Percutaneous Stellate Ganglion Block for Electrical Storm

Simone Savastano
Editor

Percutaneous Stellate Ganglion Block for Electrical Storm

Springer

Editor
Simone Savastano
Division of Cardiology
Arrhythmology and Electrophysiology Unit
Fondazione IRCCS Policlinico San Matteo
Pavia, Italy

ISBN 978-3-031-81761-8 ISBN 978-3-031-81762-5 (eBook)
https://doi.org/10.1007/978-3-031-81762-5

The publisher would like to thank Il Pensiero Scientifico for granting permission to re-use the illustrations created for the Italian edition.

Translation from the Italian language edition: “Il blocco percutaneo del ganglio stellato a scopo antiaritmico” by Simone Savastano, © Il Pensiero Scientifico 2022. Published by Il Pensiero Scientifico.

This Springer imprint is published by the registered company Springer Nature Switzerland AG
The registered company address is: Gewerbestrasse 11, 6330 Cham, Switzerland

Foreword

One of the greatest rewards of academic life is the realisation that former students and young researchers have become true colleagues and that—on their own merits—they have matured scientifically to the point of making significant contributions to the scientific literature. This is the case of Simone Savastano, a case that is plastically demonstrated by this manual, written with contributions from several of my other former students.

This manual provides all the information, theoretical and above all practical, that will allow the creation in as many cardiology departments as possible of teams capable of intervening in the not uncommon and highly dramatic cases of electrical storm by using the left stellate ganglion block. There have been a number of publications on this topic in recent years, but the work of Savastano et al. [1] represented an important step forward, both because of its anatomy-based approach without the need for echo-guidance and because of its focus on the left stellate ganglion.

Here, it is appropriate for me to make two confessions.

The first is that the brilliant results of Savastano and his collaborators are music to my ears, because since the very early 1970s, a significant part of my research, having as its primary objective the prevention of lethal arrhythmias both during acute myocardial ischaemia and in patients with long QT syndrome, was focused precisely on ablation of the left stellate ganglion to block the release of noradrenaline at the ventricular level [2, 3].

The second is that in 1975 I had written extensively *against* pharmacological blockade of the stellate ganglia [4], and I must now contradict myself, at least in part. At that time, I opposed the growing trend of pharmacological block of the stellate ganglia to assess whether it could have antiarrhythmic efficacy; this approach relied on the appearance of Horner's syndrome to assume that there was complete blockade of the stellate ganglia. My reasoning was that Horner's syndrome appears as soon as a local anaesthetic reaches the upper part of the stellate ganglion, where the fibres directed to the eye pass through, and this in itself does not necessarily imply blockage of the sympathetic fibres directed to the heart, which are located more distally. Simone Savastano's data oblige me to take a more ... open view.

In this sense, I would like to recall an episode that is quite random in itself but is directly related to the rational basis of the new therapeutic approach of Savastano and co-workers. In 1974–1975, I was working in Galveston, Texas, on my first experimental model of sudden death, based on the clinical observation that most sudden deaths occurred in patients who had a brief episode of acute myocardial ischaemia on top of a previous infarction. In the first stage, in dogs under general anaesthesia, the left descending coronary artery was occluded and an inflatable balloon was placed from the outside around the circumflex. After approximately 1–2 months—when the dogs had fully recovered and were conscious—a short occlusion of the circumflex was performed, while the left or right stellate ganglion was blocked for a few minutes by cooling. One of the problems in the laboratory was that, quite frequently, in the first hour after the creation of the anterior infarct, severe ventricular arrhythmias appeared, leading to ventricular fibrillation and loss of the animal. It was therefore imperative to try to prevent this from happening. One day it happened that, while the animal's chest was still open, ventricular arrhythmias appeared and were continually increasing, and I feared losing the dog. I decided at that point to put lidocaine on the stellate ganglion and told the technician to mark on the paper the moment I did so. The figure in (a) shows at high speed the ventricular premature beats with the impact on the tachogram; in (b), at low speed, you can see how a few minutes after blocking the nerve transmission in the stellate ganglion the ventricular arrhythmias ceased completely.

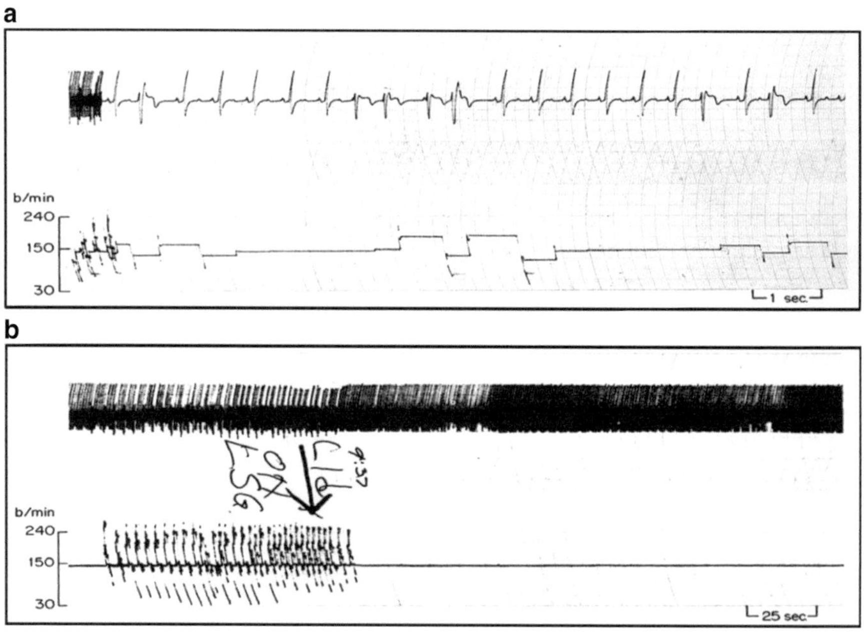

(**a**) ECG and tachogram recorded in anaesthetised dog 30 min after occlusion of the left descending coronary artery to create a myocardial infarction. Numerous ventricular premature beats appear in response to myocardial ischaemia, clearly visible on the ECG and tachogram. (**b**) Since these arrhythmias often trigger runs of ventricular tachycardia which can result in ventricular fibrillation, and since the animals had to survive the acute infarction in order to be studied about a month later, it was important to try to reduce the arrhythmias. A few drops of lidocaine directly on the left stellate ganglion (the thorax was still open) blocked nerve transmission, producing an immediate cessation of arrhythmias. This gave rise to the idea that life-threatening arrhythmias could be interrupted by injecting lidocaine into, or around, the left stellate ganglion. Clinical developments from this observation are changing the clinical approach to patients with an electrical storm (*from ref. 5*)

This simple figure, published in 1978 in my first book [5], opened the door to subsequent clinical developments and—after many years—to this very useful manual by Simone Savastano.

Centre for the Study and Treatment of Cardiac Arrhythmias of Genetic Origin
Italian Auxological Institute, IRCCS,
Milan, Italy

Peter J. Schwartz

References

1. Savastano S, Dusi V, Baldi E, Rordorf R, Sanzo A, Camporotondo R, Fracchia R, Compagnoni S, Frigerio L, Oltrona Visconti L, De Ferrari GM. Anatomical-based percutaneous left stellate ganglion block in patients with drug-refractory electrical storm and structural heart disease: a single-centre case series. Europace 2021;23:581–6.
2. Schwartz PJ. Cardiac sympathetic denervation to prevent life-threatening arrhythmias. Nat Rev Cardiol 2014;11:346–53.
3. Schwartz PJ. Cutting nerves and saving lives. Heart Rhythm 2009;6:760–3.
4. Schwartz PJ, Periti M, Malliani A. The long QT syndrome. Am Heart J 1975;89:378-90.
5. Schwartz PJ, Stone HL. Unilateral stellectomy and sudden death. In: Schwartz PJ, Brown AM, Malliani A, Zanchetti A, editors. Neural mechanisms in cardiac arrhythmias. New York: Raven Press; 1978. p. 107–22.

Preface

An electrical storm is one of the most challenging emergencies in cardiology as pharmacological treatments are few and not always effective, and non-pharmacological treatments are not widely available 24/7. So, cardiologists, intensivists, and emergency physicians may have to deal with a critical patient, burdened by a high risk of death due to recurrent ventricular arrhythmias, with a limited range of options. Such patients may need to be stabilised before being transported to centres capable of implementing non-pharmacological treatments, such as transcatheter ablation or circulatory mechanic support, or before receiving interventional treatment. Percutaneous stellate ganglion block fits perfectly into this context. In fact, this technique, developed in the first half of the 1900s for antalgic purposes, was later supported by the results of studies in the 1970s which demonstrated a central role for the autonomic nervous system in the genesis and maintenance of ventricular arrhythmias. The aim of this manual is to provide the reader with an overview of the rationale, efficacy, safety, and technique of its execution so that this procedure can be disseminated, increasing the therapeutic options for the management of patients with arrhythmic storm.

This manual will discuss many aspects useful in daily clinical practice: from the pathophysiology of ventricular arrhythmias, to the modern treatment of arrhythmic storm, to the role of the autonomic nervous system on cardiac electrophysiology and the genesis and maintenance of ventricular arrhythmias. Data available in the literature to date on the use of this technique for anti-arrhythmic purposes will be reviewed, and finally, after a due anatomical overview, the techniques for approaching the stellate ganglion will be discussed in detail both with the aid of imaging techniques and by anatomical landmarks. In this book, you will also find a reference to an instructional video that will help you learn how to perform the technique safely.

After wishing you all a good read, I would like to express a number of thanks.

My first thanks go to the *co-authors* of this manual for sharing and supporting the project and for devoting their time not only to writing but also to teaching. Disseminating an effective technique that can improve the management of complex patients like those with arrhythmic storm has been a source of great satisfaction for us.

A special thank goes to *Chiara Barbaglia* for translating most of the manual from the Italian to the English version.

I would like to thank *Prof. P.J. Schwartz*, teacher and model, for agreeing to write the preface to this manual, giving it the importance that comes from his profound experience in this field. His preface is not only a personal honour for myself but also a tribute to the thread linking his experimental experiences in the 1970s and our clinical dissemination of today.

Special thanks go to *Dr. Diego Beltrutti*, anaesthesiologist and pain therapist, who in his hospital career performed hundreds of stellate ganglion blocks by anatomical technique. He, among others, deserves the credit for teaching us the technique by anatomical landmarks alone, allowing us to extend the procedure to anti-arrhythmic purposes and to distinguish our work within an international field that still largely employs imaging aids. We believe that the technique by anatomical landmarks alone has introduced a simple and extremely versatile approach for cardiologists in the management of AS.

I would also like to thank that *IRCCS Policlinico San Matteo Foundation,* for which I have the honour to work and for supporting us in the organisation of training courses for our national and international colleagues. These have been an opportunity not only to share specific techniques and experiences but also to create a network of clinical and research purposes.

I would also like to express my heartfelt thanks to our regional emergency medical service, the *Azienda Regionale dell'emergenza-urgenza* (***AREU***) of the Lombardy Region, and in particular to our colleagues of the emergency system of the province of *Pavia. They* not only supported the organisation of the training courses and the drafting of this manual but also strongly believed in this project and helped us export it to out-of-hospital settings.

The added value of our training courses is the creation of a 3D model, specially designed and created by the clinical 3D printing laboratory "3D4Med" and hosted by the Foundation IRCCS Policlinico San Matteo in Pavia. It is the first 3D printing laboratory for clinical purposes in Italy and one of the first in the world and has allowed us to create a so-far unavailable, high-fidelity tool that can be used repeatedly for training in the stellate ganglion block with an ultrasound-guided approach. My heartfelt thanks to them.

Thanks are also due to the *Italian Association of Arrhythmology and Cardiostimulation* (*AIAC*), for giving us the opportunity to produce an instructional video, available on the AIAC YouTube channel, in which both the frontal approach technique with anatomical exhibits and the lateral ultrasound-guided approach are illustrated.

A special thanks goes to the publisher Il Pensiero Scientifico for their collaboration during the preparation of this book.

Finally, I would like to thank *all of you, the readers of* this manual, in the hope that you will find it useful and that it will provide you with a valuable support in your clinical practice.

Pavia, Italy Simone Savastano

Contents

Part I

Background

1 Ventricular Arrhythmias

Antonio Sanzo and Roberto Rordorf

Introduction

Ventricular arrhythmias (VA) include a wide spectrum ranging from premature ventricular contraction (PVC) to ventricular tachycardia (VT), ventricular fibrillation (VF), and electrical storm (ES). Their clinical presentation varies widely, from a complete lack of symptoms to the most dramatic scenario of cardiac arrest.

Ventricular tachycardia is a hyperkinetic arrhythmia characterized by three or more than three consecutive beats originating from the ventricles, distal to the His bundle. VT is defined by a heart rate between 100 and 250 bpm; if the rate is between 100 and 120 bpm, it is referred to as slow VT, while a rate greater than 250 bpm is termed ventricular flutter. VF is an absolute ventricular arrhythmia characterized by chaotic and disorganized electrical activity; on an electrocardiogram, it presents as continuous activation with varying morphology, amplitude, and direction [1]. Electrical storm is characterized by repetitive ventricular tachycardia/fibrillation (VT/VF) episodes occurring over a short period (three or more episodes within 24 hours) [2].

(translated by Chiara Barbaglia)

A. Sanzo (✉) · R. Rordorf
Division of Cardiology, Arrhythmology and Electrophysiology Unit, Fondazione IRCCS Policlinico San Matteo, Pavia, Italy
e-mail: an.sanzo@smatteo.pv.it

S. Savastano (ed.), *Percutaneous Stellate Ganglion Block for Electrical Storm*,
https://doi.org/10.1007/978-3-031-81762-5_1

Epidemiology

Ventricular tachycardia and VF account for most out-of-hospital cardiac arrest cases. The incidence of out-of-hospital arrest in people of any age is 76.5 individuals per 100,000 inhabitants/year according to the 2019 Cardiac Arrest Registry to Enhance Survival (CARES) registry, with variations between different countries (range 41.8–126.1) [3]. VAs represent about half of deaths related to cardiac causes. The risk of out-of-hospital cardiac arrest and sudden cardiac death is higher in men than in women and increases with age due to the higher prevalence of ischemic heart disease in older age [4].

In about half of patients with out-of-hospital cardiac arrest and presenting rhythm identified as VF, the underlying cause of cardiac arrest is acute myocardial infarction. Of all out-of-hospital cardiac arrests, more than 50% have significant coronary lesions at primary coronary angiography [5]. Sustained VAs occurring during acute coronary syndromes (ACS) are more often polymorphic VT or VF rather than monomorphic VT.

Patients with structural heart disease are at increased risk of sustained VT and VF. Sustained VT not associated with ACS is predominantly monomorphic as it is frequently due to an anatomical reentry mechanism related to a scar or functional block. However, even monomorphic VT in the context of chronic ischemic heart disease can degenerate into VF. Monomorphic VT occurring in the absence of structural heart disease is commonly referred to as idiopathic VT and is often due to increased automaticity. Polymorphic VT and VF occurring in the absence of structural heart disease are rare and may be due to channelopathies [6], drug-induced long QT syndrome [7], or may be idiopathic [8]. VT is rare in children but can occur in the presence of structural heart disease. Overall, VT is more common in men than in women [4].

Classification

The 2006 American College of Cardiology/American Heart Association Task Force on Clinical Data Standards Report classifies VTs based on clinical characteristics, morphology, duration, and pathophysiological mechanism [1].

Clinically, VT can be hemodynamically stable if it does not compromise vital functions or hemodynamically unstable when it causes hemodynamic compromise (hypotension, angina, dyspnea, loss of consciousness) and requires prompt interruption. A VT can initially be hemodynamically tolerated but may cause progressive hemodynamic deterioration once compensatory mechanisms are exhausted.

VTs are defined as idiopathic in the absence of known underlying heart disease, or they are associated with chronic or acute heart conditions (infarction or myocarditis) or channelopathies.

The classification of VTs depends on duration and morphology (Table 1.1). Non-sustained ventricular tachycardia (NSVT) is defined as more than three beats at a

Table 1.1 Definitions

Clinical characteristics
• Hemodynamically stable
• Hemodynamically unstable
• Idiopathic
• Associated with a chronic cardiomyopathy
• Associated with an acute event
• Associated with channelopathy
• Ventricular ectopic beat
• Non-sustained ventricular tachycardia
• Sustained ventricular tachycardia
• Incessant ventricular tachycardia
• Repetitive ventricular tachycardia
• Electrical storm
Underlying mechanism
• Focal ventricular tachycardia
• Reentrant ventricular tachycardia
– Scar related
– Functional
Morphological characteristics
Monomorphic ventricular tachycardia
Polymorphic ventricular tachycardia
Pleiomorphic ventricular tachycardia
Torsades de pointes

rate greater than 100 bpm lasting less than 30 s. When VT lasts more than 30 s or hemodynamic instability occurs in less than 30 s, it is considered sustained VT. VAs can be incessant when they do not terminate despite pharmacological and instrumental interventions or repetitive if they stop and restart. Electrical storm is defined as three or more episodes of sustained VA occurring within a 24-h period [2]. This definition is widely adopted, as it is clinically significant and related to worse short- and long-term outcomes [9].

Morphologically, VTs are classified as monomorphic (stable QRS beat to beat), polymorphic (variable and multiform QRS beat to beat), pleomorphic (during the same VT episode, there are multiple monomorphic forms, with QRS stabilizing in different), or with multiple morphologies (distinct VT episodes with different QRS morphologies). Torsades de pointes is a polymorphic VT occurring in the context of congenital or acquired long QT syndrome, characterized electrocardiographically by twisting of the QRS complexes around the isoelectric line with progressively increasing and decreasing QRS amplitude. Bidirectional VT is defined by the alternation of the QRS axis in the frontal plane beat to beat; it is associated with digitalis toxicity or catecholaminergic polymorphic VT.

VT is termed focal or micro-reentrant when ventricular activation originates from a pinpoint area in the ventricle and spreads to other regions or reentrant/macro-reentrant when the activation circuit revolves around an area of anatomical or functional block.

Mechanisms

The three common mechanisms underlying all arrhythmias are increased ectopic automaticity, afterdepolarizations (early and delayed), and reentry circuits.

Increased automaticity is related to spontaneous depolarizations originating from damaged or abnormally excitable tissue, which is normally activated by the wave front of regular ventricular depolarization. Increased ventricular automaticity occurs more frequently in Purkinje fibers. These normally quiescent fibers, when partially depolarized (such as during ischemia), can progressively depolarize during phase 4 of the action potential until reaching the threshold for triggering a new action potential. The spontaneous activation of Purkinje fibers is linked to the activation of the I_f current, which becomes active between −90 and −60 mV, making it more frequent during ischemia. Catecholamines shorten the action potential and promote phase 4 depolarization, especially when associated with other factors such as hypokalemia; this can facilitate VAs, including VF.

Afterdepolarizations are associated with alterations in ionic currents and transmembrane electrical homeostasis. Delayed afterdepolarizations (DADs) are oscillations in phase 4 of the action potential which, if reaching the threshold, can trigger a new action potential. DADs are linked to cytoplasmic calcium overload, which promotes sodium entry into the cell through the sodium–calcium exchanger. DADs are favored by high heart rates, adrenergic activation, and factors such as digitalis intoxication. Tachycardia and heart failure lead to shortening of the action potential duration and intracellular calcium overload, facilitating the onset of VAs.

Early afterdepolarizations (EADs) occur during the plateau phase (phase 2) or repolarization phase (phase 3) of the action potential. EADs are often associated with bradycardia, ischemia, and congenital or induced ion channel disorders. The sodium–calcium exchanger current is believed to play a key role in the development of EADs. A significant predisposing factor is calcium overload, which can occur in heart failure with excessive adrenergic stimulation that increases calcium entry via the sodium–calcium exchanger. Arrhythmias associated with EADs more frequently include early extrasystoles (R-on-T phenomenon), torsades de pointes, and VF.

Reentry circuits are based on the dispersion of action potential duration and refractoriness, with nonhomogeneous electrical activation of the ventricular myocardium. Ischemia, electrolyte imbalances, fibrosis, sympathetic hyperactivity, cellular uncoupling, and electrolyte imbalance favor the dispersion of refractoriness. Reentry circuits can be micro-reentries (the circuit, predominantly functional, is anchored to a circumscribed region with very short action potential duration) or macro-reentries around an anatomical scar or a region of functional block. Stable anatomical reentry circuits around a scar underlie sustained VTs. A non-excitable post-infarction scar or a large vessel like the aorta or the right ventricular outflow tract can form a pathway for a stable reentrant circuit. Functional conduction blocks can also occur without an anatomical non-excitable core. Large reentrant circuits involving the entire ventricle can form, especially in cardiomyopathies with severe ventricular dilation and/or significant intramuscular conduction slowing.

VF is frequently secondary to the degeneration of a VT. VT is favored by substrate changes that facilitate focal activity or reentry. Variations in conduction velocity and refractoriness dispersion can lead to the degeneration of VT into VF. The mechanisms of ventricular fibrillation are multiple reentries (wavelet reentry) or a rotor that fractionates and breaks into multiple wave fronts.

Electrical storm is frequently secondary to monomorphic VTs in structural heart disease with a reentry mechanism related to a scar [10]. The conduction system, particularly the Purkinje fibers, can serve as a substrate for electrical storm secondary to monomorphic VTs, usually in the context of concomitant structural heart disease [11, 12].

Electrical storm secondary to polymorphic VT or VF generally develops in acute myocardial infarction and advanced heart failure, in arrhythmogenic inherited cardiomyopathy, and in a wide range of structural heart anomalies or channelopathies. Arrhythmias are often sustained by functional reentry [13]. Purkinje fibers commonly originate the triggers for electrical storm characterized by polymorphic VT and VF in acute myocardial ischemia [14].

Physiopathology of Ventricular Arrhythmias

The heart is an electrically and hemodynamically stable structure, with mechanisms ensuring homeostasis and the ability to compensate for sudden rhythm and mechanical disturbances. It also possesses the capacity for remodeling and regeneration. The onset of sustained VA results from a complex interaction between pre-existing pathological conditions that create a vulnerable substrate, dynamic modulation factors such as myocardial ischemia and changes in autonomic tone, and specific triggers (specific to each heart disease). The substrate, the modulating factor, and the triggering factor play a fundamental role in the onset and maintenance of VT/VF. They act synergistically by increasing or triggering abnormal automaticity of myocardial cells and/or promoting dispersion and therefore reentry circuits (Fig. 1.1).

The term *substrate* refers to the presence of a pre-existing cardiac abnormality that increases the likelihood of reentry. Although there are cases of idiopathic VAs (i.e., without an evident substrate), a structural anomaly is often necessary for the initiation and perpetuation of a VA. The substrate can be myocardial structural (e.g., post-myocardial infarction scars, myocarditis, hypertrophy, or dilation), coronary, electrical (at the anatomical level, such as Wolff–Parkinson–White syndrome, more often at the channel level, such as long QT syndrome or Brugada syndrome), or nervous.

The most typical substrate alteration is a previous myocardial infarction; other diseases that predispose to VAs include hypertrophic cardiomyopathy, dilated cardiomyopathy, arrhythmogenic cardiomyopathy, congenital anomalies (e.g., an anomalous origin of the coronary arteries), and coronary spasm. Acute myocardial damage (acute infarction, myocarditis, drugs) can significantly affect the electrical dispersion of the substrate, promoting arrhythmias.

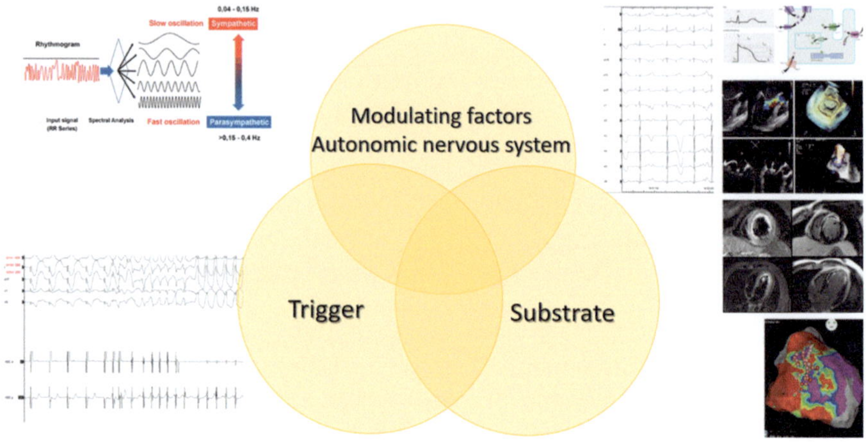

Fig. 1.1 The interaction between modulation mechanisms, triggering factors, and substrate forms the foundation of the pathophysiology of ventricular arrhythmia

Structural heart diseases involve pathological changes, including diffuse fibrosis, fat deposition, discrete scars, and alterations in electrophysiological properties caused by ion channel remodeling, providing a substrate for focal and/or reentrant VT [15].

Structural alterations have recently been implicated as a substrate for VF associated with Brugada syndrome (BrS), early repolarization syndrome (ERS), and idiopathic VF [16]. The primary arrhythmogenic substrate in BrS is believed to be localized in the epicardium of the right ventricular outflow tract, where marked interstitial myocardial fibrosis is present [17]. However, there is also substantial evidence for a central role of transmural repolarization gradients [18]. Epicardial regions hosting late depolarization anomalies or abnormal electrograms (mainly on the epicardial surface) have also been found in a subset of patients with ERS (with or without BrS characteristics) or idiopathic VF [19, 20] (Fig. 1.2).

The nervous substrate plays a fundamental role in the genesis of arrhythmias. Cardiac innervation is plastic both centrally and peripherally. Remodeling is triggered by structural alterations, muscle remodeling, and cardiac fibrosis. Myocardial infarction causes the death of sympathetic fibers within the scar and the loss of efferent sympathetic innervation in peri-scar non-infarcted sites. Noradrenaline depletion in the scar is accompanied by increased production in peri-scar non-infarcted areas. Denervated areas show supersensitivity to denervation, defined as an exaggerated response to noradrenaline infusion. Transmural myocardial infarction and heart failure can not only alter the myocardial substrate for arrhythmias but also disrupt the innervation of histologically viable myocardium, leading to supersensitivity and a nonuniform electrophysiological response to sympathetic stimulation. This contributes to generating the substrate for VAs in both acute and chronic myocardial infarction.

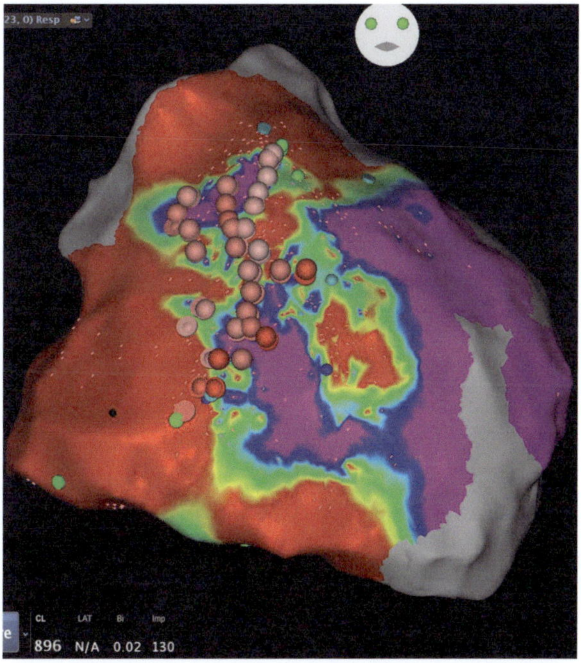

Fig. 1.2 Electroanatomic epicardial mapping in a patient with Brugada syndrome. Red areas represent regions with low-voltage EGM consistent with an electrically altered substratum

In addition to acute denervation, reinnervation (nerve sprouting) and heterogeneous hyperinnervation have been observed in models of chronic myocardial infarction and heart failure. Peripheral nerve injury, resulting in Wallerian degeneration, leads to increased nerve growth factor (NGF), which triggers nerve regeneration. Reinnervation, predominantly in peri-scar and perivascular regions, is heterogeneous, favoring electrical dispersion and consequently increasing the risk of VT and VF.

Beyond cardiac neural remodeling, extracardiac neural remodeling has also been described. In the context of myocardial infarction and heart failure, electroanatomical remodeling of the left stellate ganglion has been demonstrated: increased stellate ganglion activity immediately after infarction, associated with intramyocardial nerve sprouting, as well as increased neuronal size and synaptic density in both the left and right stellate ganglia [21]. In human cadavers with cardiac scars, the number and size of neurons in the left stellate ganglion are increased compared to cadavers without scars [22]. Similarly, compared to cadavers with normal hearts, those with cardiomyopathy show increased neuronal size and synaptophysin density [23]. These findings provide a possible mechanistic link between intramyocardial neural remodeling, stellate ganglion remodeling, and VAs. The interaction between denervated areas, regional nerve sprouting, neural remodeling, electrical remodeling due to heart failure, and electroanatomical remodeling of the stellate ganglia combine to create a substrate that favors malignant VAs (Fig. 1.3).

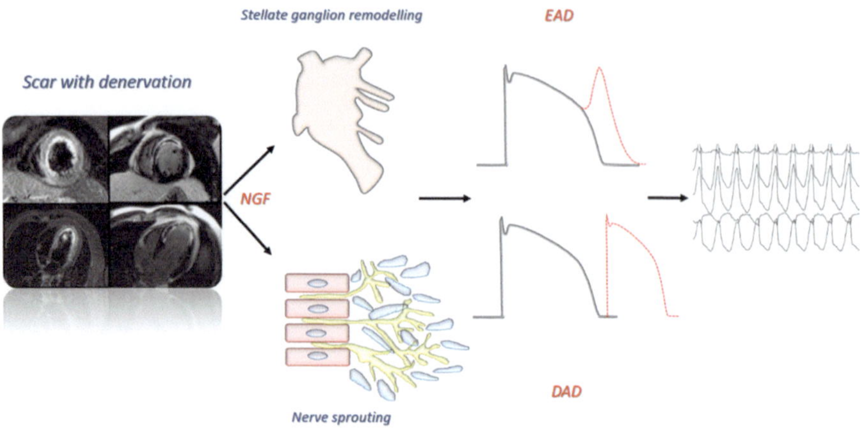

Fig. 1.3 Both central and peripheral neural remodeling are triggered by structural alterations through the increase of nerve growth factor (NGF). Nerve sprouting, heterogeneous hyperinnervation, and stellate ganglion remodeling promote early depolarizations and the occurrence of ventricular arrhythmias

Furthermore, heart failure causes remodeling of cardiac ion channels, including increased density of L-type calcium channels (I_{CaL}), decreased potassium current, reduced density of I_{to}, and alterations in chloride and calcium channels [24–27].

The onset and type of the most frequent VA correlate with the arrhythmic substrate. In the presence of a myocardial substrate that favors the formation of reentry circuits (e.g., fibrosis in patients with previous infarction or arrhythmogenic dysplasia), the most common initial arrhythmic mechanism is monomorphic VT arising without transient myocardial ischemia. In acute myocardial ischemia, the immediate onset of VF is significantly more frequent, often triggered by an early ventricular extrasystole falling just before the peak of the T wave (R-on-T phenomenon). In heart failure patients, the most common VA is polymorphic VT, typically rapidly degenerating into VF. In patients with long QT syndrome (congenital and acquired), the most typical arrhythmia is torsades de pointes tachycardia with degeneration into VF. In rare cases, VF is triggered by atrial fibrillation conducted to the ventricle via an accessory pathway with extremely low refractoriness.

The *triggering factor* is the event that destabilizes homeostasis. The most important triggering factor is an acute ischemic episode. Pathological observations of patients who died suddenly suggest that the pathophysiology of sudden death often shares characteristics with other acute cardiac events, such as the unstable phase of angina. Autopsies of suddenly deceased patients may reveal both occlusive coronary lesions, as seen in acute myocardial infarction, and nonocclusive lesions, suggesting that transient myocardial ischemia often causes sudden cardiac death. Supporting this hypothesis is the fact that only a portion of patients resuscitated after cardiac arrest develop classic myocardial infarction with ST-segment elevation. Myocardial ischemia increases myocardial electrical dispersion, associated with increased automaticity and early or delayed afterdepolarizations, and promotes the reentry mechanism [28].

Frequent ventricular extrasystoles have traditionally been considered an important triggering factor. This hypothesis originated from the observation that frequent ventricular extrasystoles on 24-hour electrocardiograms, performed on patients with a history of recent or past myocardial infarction, identified patients with higher mortality [29]. This predictive value was later confirmed in revascularized patients [30]. Therefore, it was suggested that pharmacologically abolishing the triggering factor could reduce arrhythmic mortality.

Although focal excitation due to increased automaticity or triggered activity can trigger VT, frequent ventricular extrasystoles alone are insufficient to trigger VAs. The theory that ventricular extrasystoles alone are the triggering factor was challenged by data from the CAST study, which showed that using an antiarrhythmic drug that almost eliminated ventricular extrasystoles was associated with a significant increase in cardiac mortality post-myocardial infarction [31]. These results underscore the difference between the etiopathogenesis of malignant arrhythmias underlying sudden cardiac death and that of ventricular extrasystoles. The triggering of VAs depends on the synergistic action of triggering and modulating factors on a predisposed substrate. Drugs used to reduce ventricular extrasystoles increased repolarization dispersion by further slowing conduction in the scar, creating a substrate that favored reentrant VAs. The effect of reducing the potential triggering factor was nullified by the effect on the substrate. Therefore, frequent ventricular extrasystoles should be considered an epiphenomenon and a risk marker rather than a cause or strict triggering factor.

In inherited arrhythmogenic diseases, triggering factors are events that cause action potential disturbances, initiating afterdepolarizations and leading to triggered activity, which is the triggering mechanism for torsades de pointes [32].

The term *modulating factor* refers to a time-variable factor that, under certain circumstances, can favor the onset, perpetuation, or degeneration of a ventricular arrhythmia. Typical examples include electrolyte disturbances such as hypokalemia (less commonly hypomagnesemia), which occur frequently, particularly in patients undergoing chronic diuretic therapy. Other possibilities include transient situations of hypoxia or acidosis or the use of drugs with potential proarrhythmic effects.

The autonomic nervous system has assumed a primary importance among the modulating factors of VAs and electrical storms. Numerous experimental studies have indicated the unfavorable effect of excessive sympathetic activation in the genesis of malignant ventricular arrhythmias, particularly during acute myocardial ischemia. Excessive adrenergic activation exerts several unfavorable effects, including increasing the severity of ischemia (due to increased oxygen consumption and coronary resistance), increasing the likelihood of unidirectional conduction block, and triggering arrhythmias through altered automaticity. Parasympathetic activation has often been shown to effectively counteract the unfavorable effects of increased adrenergic activation [33].

In the Temperature-Related Incidence of Electrical Storm (TEMPEST) study on 246 patients with electrical storm, 83% of whom had cardiomyopathy, the prevalence of electrical storm was significantly higher on workdays and during daytime hours [33].

Significant associations between stressful global events and cardiac arrest statistics have also been reported [34]. Additionally, arrhythmic events in long QT syndrome (LQTS) types 1 and 2 and catecholaminergic polymorphic VT (CPVT) are often induced by physical or emotional stress. Sympathetic hyperactivity after ICD discharge can trigger further tachyarrhythmias, occasionally initiating electrical storms in patients with ICD for CPVT or (more rarely) LQTS [35]. In contrast, the onset of arrhythmias in BrS, ERS, short QT syndrome, and idiopathic ventricular fibrillation usually occurs during sleep or rest, conditions associated with high parasympathetic tone [36].

Many studies have suggested that sympathetic nerve stimulation, particularly left stellate ganglion (LSG) stimulation, is proarrhythmic. LSG stimulation has been observed to cause greater increases in early afterdepolarization amplitude [37].

Sympathetic stimulation affects the action potential and restitution, which, along with increased I_{CaL} density, can lead to afterdepolarizations induced by intracellular Ca^{2+} overload, enhancing the risk of spontaneous ventricular arrhythmias. Additionally, sympathetic stimulation increases refractoriness dispersion by shortening refractoriness in nonischemic sites without changing or increasing refractoriness in ischemic sites [38].

References

1. Buxton AE, Calkins H, Callans DJ, DiMarco JP, Fisher JD, Greene HL, Haines DE, Hayes DL, Heidenreich PA, Miller JM, et al. ACC/AHA/HRS 2006 key data elements and definitions for electrophysiological studies and procedures: a report of the American College of Cardiology/American Heart Association Task Force on Clinical Data Standards (ACC/AHA/HRS Writing Committee to Develop Data Standards on Electrophysiology). Circulation. 2006;114:2534–70. https://doi.org/10.1161/CIRCULATIONAHA.106.180199.
2. Credner SC, Klingenheben T, Mauss O, Sticherling C, Hohnloser SH. Electrical storm in patients with transvenous implantable cardioverter-defibrillators: incidence, management and prognostic implications. J Am Coll Cardiol. 1998;32:1909–15. https://doi.org/10.1016/s0735-1097(98)00495-1.
3. Virani SS, Alonso A, Aparicio HJ, Benjamin EJ, Bittencourt MS, Callaway CW, Carson AP, Chamberlain AM, Cheng S, Delling FN, et al. Heart disease and stroke statistics-2021 update: a report from the American Heart Association. Circulation. 2021;143:e254–743. https://doi.org/10.1161/CIR.0000000000000950.
4. Priori SG, Blomström-Lundqvist C, Mazzanti A, Blom N, Borggrefe M, Camm J, Elliott PM, Fitzsimons D, Hatala R, Hindricks G, et al. 2015 ESC guidelines for the management of patients with ventricular arrhythmias and the prevention of sudden cardiac death: the task force for the management of patients with ventricular arrhythmias and the prevention of sudden cardiac death of the European Society of Cardiology (ESC). Endorsed by: Association for European Paediatric and Congenital Cardiology (AEPC). Eur Heart J. 2015;36:2793–867. https://doi.org/10.1093/eurheartj/ehv316.
5. Dumas F, Cariou A, Manzo-Silberman S, Grimaldi D, Vivien B, Rosencher J, Empana JP, Carli P, Mira JP, Jouven X, Spaulding C. Immediate percutaneous coronary intervention is associated with better survival after out-of-hospital cardiac arrest: insights from the PROCAT (Parisian region out of hospital cardiac ArresT) registry. Circ Cardiovasc Interv. 2010;3:200–7. https://doi.org/10.1161/CIRCINTERVENTIONS.109.913665.

6. Ackerman MJ, Priori SG, Willems S, Berul C, Brugada R, Calkins H, Camm AJ, Ellinor PT, Gollob M, Hamilton R, et al. HRS/EHRA expert consensus statement on the state of genetic testing for the channelopathies and cardiomyopathies: this document was developed as a partnership between the Heart Rhythm Society (HRS) and the European Heart Rhythm Association (EHRA). Europace. 2011;13:1077–109. https://doi.org/10.1093/europace/eur245.
7. Nannenberg EA, Sijbrands EJ, Dijksman LM, Alders M, van Tintelen JP, Birnie M, van Langen IM, Wilde AA. Mortality of inherited arrhythmia syndromes: insight into their natural history. Circ Cardiovasc Genet. 2012;5:183–9. https://doi.org/10.1161/CIRCGENETICS.111.961102.
8. Haïssaguerre M, Shah DC, Jaïs P, Shoda M, Kautzner J, Arentz T, Kalushe D, Kadish A, Griffith M, Gaïta F, et al. Role of Purkinje conducting system in triggering of idiopathic ventricular fibrillation. Lancet. 2002;359:677–8. https://doi.org/10.1016/S0140-6736(02)07807-8.
9. Exner DV, Pinski SL, Wyse DG, Renfroe EG, Follmann D, Gold M, Beckman KJ, Coromilas J, Lancaster S, Hallstrom AP, Defibrillators AIAVI. Electrical storm presages nonsudden death: the antiarrhythmics versus implantable defibrillators (AVID) trial. Circulation. 2001;103:2066–71. https://doi.org/10.1161/01.cir.103.16.2066.
10. Nayyar S, Ganesan AN, Brooks AG, Sullivan T, Roberts-Thomson KC, Sanders P. Venturing into ventricular arrhythmia storm: a systematic review and meta-analysis. Eur Heart J. 2013;34:560–71. https://doi.org/10.1093/eurheartj/ehs453.
11. Hayashi M, Kobayashi Y, Iwasaki YK, Morita N, Miyauchi Y, Kato T, Takano T. Novel mechanism of postinfarction ventricular tachycardia originating in surviving left posterior Purkinje fibers. Heart Rhythm. 2006;3:908–18. https://doi.org/10.1016/j.hrthm.2006.04.019.
12. Reithmann C, Hahnefeld A, Ulbrich M, Matis T, Steinbeck G. Different forms of ventricular tachycardia involving the left anterior fascicle in nonischemic cardiomyopathy: critical sites of the reentrant circuit in low-voltage areas. J Cardiovasc Electrophysiol. 2009;20:841–9. https://doi.org/10.1111/j.1540-8167.2009.01467.x.
13. Majumder R, Nayak AR, Pandit R. Scroll-wave dynamics in human cardiac tissue: lessons from a mathematical model with inhomogeneities and fiber architecture. PLoS One. 2011;6:e18052. https://doi.org/10.1371/journal.pone.0018052.
14. Komatsu Y, Hocini M, Nogami A, Maury P, Peichl P, Iwasaki YK, Masuda K, Denis A, Voglimacci-Stephanopoli Q, Wichterle D, et al. Catheter ablation of refractory ventricular fibrillation storm after myocardial infarction. Circulation. 2019;139:2315–25. https://doi.org/10.1161/CIRCULATIONAHA.118.037997.
15. Nattel S, Maguy A, Le Bouter S, Yeh YH. Arrhythmogenic ion-channel remodeling in the heart: heart failure, myocardial infarction, and atrial fibrillation. Physiol Rev. 2007;87:425–56. https://doi.org/10.1152/physrev.00014.2006.
16. Haïssaguerre M, Duchateau J, Dubois R, Hocini M, Cheniti G, Sacher F, Lavergne T, Probst V, Surget E, Vigmond E, et al. Idiopathic ventricular fibrillation: role of Purkinje system and microstructural myocardial abnormalities. JACC Clin Electrophysiol. 2020;6:591–608. https://doi.org/10.1016/j.jacep.2020.03.010.
17. Nademanee K. Radiofrequency ablation in Brugada syndrome. Heart Rhythm. 2021;18:1805–6. https://doi.org/10.1016/j.hrthm.2021.08.005.
18. Antzelevitch C. Genetic, molecular and cellular mechanisms underlying the J wave syndromes. Circ J. 2012;76:1054–65. https://doi.org/10.1253/circj.cj-12-0284.
19. Nademanee K, Haissaguerre M, Hocini M, Nogami A, Cheniti G, Duchateau J, Behr ER, Saba M, Bokan R, Lou Q, et al. Mapping and ablation of ventricular fibrillation associated with early repolarization syndrome. Circulation. 2019;140:1477–90. https://doi.org/10.1161/CIRCULATIONAHA.118.039022.
20. Haïssaguerre M, Hocini M, Cheniti G, Duchateau J, Sacher F, Puyo S, Cochet H, Takigawa M, Denis A, Martin R, et al. Localized structural alterations underlying a subset of unexplained sudden cardiac death. Circ Arrhythm Electrophysiol. 2018;11:e006120. https://doi.org/10.1161/CIRCEP.117.006120.

21. Zhou S, Chen LS, Miyauchi Y, Miyauchi M, Kar S, Kangavari S, Fishbein MC, Sharifi B, Chen PS. Mechanisms of cardiac nerve sprouting after myocardial infarction in dogs. Circ Res. 2004;95:76–83. https://doi.org/10.1161/01.RES.0000133678.22968.e3.
22. Wood A, Docimo S, Elkowitz DE. Cardiovascular disease and its association with histological changes of the left stellate ganglion. Clin Med Insights Pathol. 2010;3:19–24. https://doi.org/10.4137/cpath.s4285.
23. Ajijola OA, Wisco JJ, Lambert HW, Mahajan A, Stark E, Fishbein MC, Shivkumar K. Extracardiac neural remodeling in humans with cardiomyopathy. Circ Arrhythm Electrophysiol. 2012;5:1010–116. https://doi.org/10.1161/CIRCEP.112.972836.
24. Huang B, Qin D, El-Sherif N. Early down-regulation of K+ channel genes and currents in the postinfarction heart. J Cardiovasc Electrophysiol. 2000;11:1252–61. https://doi.org/10.1046/j.1540-8167.2000.01252.x.
25. Gidh-Jain M, Huang B, Jain P, el-Sherif N. Differential expression of voltage-gated K+ channel genes in left ventricular remodeled myocardium after experimental myocardial infarction. Circ Res. 1996;79:669–75. https://doi.org/10.1161/01.res.79.4.669.
26. Qin D, Zhang ZH, Caref EB, Boutjdir M, Jain P, el-Sherif, N. Cellular and ionic basis of arrhythmias in postinfarction remodeled ventricular myocardium. Circ Res. 1996;79:461–73. https://doi.org/10.1161/01.res.79.3.461.
27. Heath BM, Xia J, Dong E, An RH, Brooks A, Liang C, Federoff HJ, Kass RS. Overexpression of nerve growth factor in the heart alters ion channel activity and beta-adrenergic signalling in an adult transgenic mouse. J Physiol. 1998;512(Pt 3):779–91. https://doi.org/10.1111/j.1469-7793.1998.779bd.x.
28. Cherry EM, Fenton FH, Gilmour RF. Mechanisms of ventricular arrhythmias: a dynamical systems-based perspective. Am J Physiol Heart Circ Physiol. 2012;302:H2451–63. https://doi.org/10.1152/ajpheart.00770.2011.
29. Bigger JT, Fleiss JL, Kleiger R, Miller JP, Rolnitzky LM. The relationships among ventricular arrhythmias, left ventricular dysfunction, and mortality in the 2 years after myocardial infarction. Circulation. 1984;69:250–8. https://doi.org/10.1161/01.cir.69.2.250.
30. Maggioni AP, Zuanetti G, Franzosi MG, Rovelli F, Santoro E, Staszewsky L, Tavazzi L, Tognoni G. Prevalence and prognostic significance of ventricular arrhythmias after acute myocardial infarction in the fibrinolytic era. GISSI-2 results. Circulation. 1993;87:312–22. https://doi.org/10.1161/01.cir.87.2.312.
31. Echt DS, Liebson PR, Mitchell LB, Peters RW, Obias-Manno D, Barker AH, Arensberg D, Baker A, Friedman L, Greene HL. Mortality and morbidity in patients receiving encainide, flecainide, or placebo. The Cardiac Arrhythmia Suppression Trial. N Engl J Med. 1991;324:781–8. https://doi.org/10.1056/NEJM199103213241201.
32. Antzelevitch C. Cellular basis and mechanism underlying normal and abnormal myocardial repolarization and arrhythmogenesis. Ann Med. 2004;36(Suppl 1):5–14. https://doi.org/10.1080/17431380410032553.
33. Guerra F, Bonelli P, Flori M, Cipolletta L, Carbucicchio C, Izquierdo M, Kozluk E, Shivkumar K, Vaseghi M, Patani F, et al. Temporal trends and temperature-related incidence of electrical storm: the TEMPEST study (temperature-related incidence of electrical storm). Circ Arrhythm Electrophysiol. 2017;10 https://doi.org/10.1161/CIRCEP.116.004634.
34. Muller A, Dyson K, Bernard S, Smith K. Seasonal variation in out-of-hospital cardiac arrest in Victoria 2008–2017: winter peak. Prehosp Emerg Care. 2020;24:769–77. https://doi.org/10.1080/10903127.2019.1708518.
35. Tsuji Y, Heijman J, Nattel S, Dobrev D. Electrical storm: recent pathophysiological insights and therapeutic consequences. Basic Res Cardiol. 2013;108:336. https://doi.org/10.1007/s00395-013-0336-2.

36. Steinberg C, Davies B, Mellor G, Tadros R, Laksman ZW, Roberts JD, Green M, Alqarawi W, Angaran P, Healey J, et al. Short-coupled ventricular fibrillation represents a distinct phenotype among latent causes of unexplained cardiac arrest: a report from the CASPER registry. Eur Heart J. 2021;42:2827–38. https://doi.org/10.1093/eurheartj/ehab275.
37. Ben-David J, Zipes DP. Differential response to right and left ansae subclaviae stimulation of early afterdepolarizations and ventricular tachycardia induced by cesium in dogs. Circulation. 1988;78:1241–50. https://doi.org/10.1161/01.cir.78.5.1241.
38. Swissa M, Zhou S, Gonzalez-Gomez I, Chang CM, Lai AC, Cates AW, Fishbein MC, Karagueuzian HS, Chen PS, Chen LS. Long-term subthreshold electrical stimulation of the left stellate ganglion and a canine model of sudden cardiac death. J Am Coll Cardiol. 2004;43:858–64. https://doi.org/10.1016/j.jacc.2003.07.053.

The Ventricular Electrical Storm

2

Roberto Rordorf and Antonio Sanzo

Definition and Prognosis

Electrical storm (ES) is a clinical emergency characterised by a cluster of ventricular arrhythmias occurring over a certain time. The two significant variables in defining an electrical storm are the number of ventricular arrhythmias and the timeframe during which they occur. The most widely used definition to date is the occurrence of three or more separate episodes of sustained ventricular arrhythmias within 24 hours.

Other criteria have been used in the past (i.e. the occurrence of two or more episodes of ventricular arrhythmias within 1 h; the occurrence of two or more defibrillator shocks within 24 h; the occurrence of 20 ventricular arrhythmias within 24 h or of 4 episodes within 1 h [1]); however, the definition based on the occurrence of three or more episodes of sustained ventricular arrhythmias in 24 h is the most widely used and accepted as its significant prognostic value has been largely demonstrated [2].

The different definitions of the clinical emergency and the variety of populations analysed make it difficult to estimate correctly the incidence of electrical storm in the general population. Considering the number of implantable defibrillator recipients, an electrical storm occurs in approximately 10–20% of cases, with a higher incidence in subjects implanted in secondary prevention as compared to patients implanted with a primary prevention indication. Electrical storm is associated with a significant worsening of prognosis, with a 2.5-fold higher risk of short-term mortality compared to patients with isolated ventricular arrhythmias and a 3.3-fold higher risk when compared to patients without ventricular arrhythmias [3].

(translated by Chiara Barbaglia)

R. Rordorf (✉) · A. Sanzo
Division of Cardiology, Arrhythmology and Electrophysiology Unit, Fondazione IRCCS Policlinico San Matteo, Pavia, Italy
e-mail: r.rordorf@smatteo.pv.it

S. Savastano (ed.), *Percutaneous Stellate Ganglion Block for Electrical Storm*, https://doi.org/10.1007/978-3-031-81762-5_2

In their study of 2020, Elsokkari et al. showed how patients presenting with recurrence of ventricular arrhythmias, even if not in the form of electrical storm, have a significantly worse prognosis [4]. These data suggest the need to classify as "high-risk patients" all patients with recurrent ventricular arrhythmias or electrical storm. In these cases, every effort should be made to remove the possible underlying causes and prevent arrhythmic recurrences. Ischaemic and nonischaemic structural heart disease are the most frequent substrates of electrical storm. Cases of electrical storm in patients with hereditary nonstructural arrhythmogenic disease—as Brugada syndrome, long QT syndrome and catecholaminergic polymorphic tachycardia—are rarer. In a low percentage of electrical storms, precise triggers could be acute ischaemia, electrolyte imbalance, worsening of heart failure or bradycardia [5].

Activation of the autonomic nervous system plays a well-recognised role in favouring the onset and the perpetuation of an electrical storm, and this may account for the higher incidence of electrical storms during working days and daylight hours [6].

The clinical presentation in a patient without a defibrillator depends on the haemodynamic tolerability of the presenting arrhythmia. In case of haemodynamic impairment, the clinical picture may be characterised by recurrent syncope or cardiac arrest; if the arrhythmia is haemodynamically well tolerated, the patient may present with palpitations or worsening heart failure. In patients with defibrillator, the clinical scenario is usually dominated by the presence of multiple defibrillator interventions such as shock or anti-tachycardia pacing (ATP). In any case, the electrical storm is a true medical emergency, requiring prompt and appropriate treatment and a multidisciplinary approach, including both pharmacological and non-pharmacological therapies (Fig. 2.1).

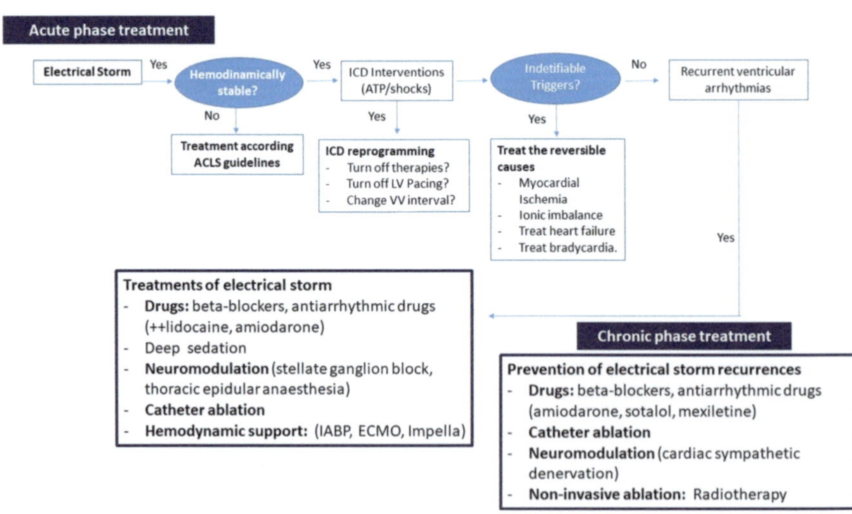

Fig. 2.1 Flowchart of electrical storm treatment. *ACLS* advanced cardiac life support, *VV delay* intraventricular delay, *IABP* intra-aortic balloon pump, *ECMO* extracorporeal membrane oxygenation

Treatment of Electrical Storm

The timely treatment of electrical storm is crucial for its short- and long-term prognosis. To date, the available treatments have not achieved satisfactory success owing to the kaleidoscopic presentation of the patient with electrical storm: substrate, modulating and triggering factors, which contribute to the onset and maintenance of the arrhythmia, are multiple and of various relevance. The lack of a widely effective treatment imposes an ongoing effort to understand the pathophysiology and treatment of electrical storm.

Pharmacological Treatment

Beta-Blockers

Activation of the sympathetic nervous system plays a central role in the initiation and maintenance of an electrical storm; for this reason, beta-blockers are determinant in the pharmacological treatment. Given the possible negative haemodynamic and inotropic effects of beta-blockers, they should be recommended with caution in patients with haemodynamic impairment or heart failure.

The first data on the use of beta-blockers in electrical storm come from a study by Nademanee et al. who randomised 49 patients with electrical storm treated with a sympathetic block therapy (propranolol, esmolol or left stellate ganglion blockade) vs. a conventional anti-arrhythmic treatment (lidocaine, procainamide or bretylium). In patients treated with sympathetic block therapy, a significant reduction in all-cause mortality was observed when compared to patients treated with anti-arrhythmic therapy [7]. In a more recent study, in a population of patients with electrical storm, the use of a nonselective beta-blocker (propranolol) proved to be more effective than the use of a β1-selective drug (metoprolol), demonstrating the importance of a nonselective blockade of the sympathetic nervous system in interrupting the vicious cycle of arrhythmogenesis [8]. However, nonselective beta-blockers can cause worsening of haemodynamic conditions in patients with severe left and/or right ventricular dysfunction and in patients with heart failure. In these cases, the use of a selective, short half-life beta-blocker—such as esmolol or landiolol—may be considered [9].

Amiodarone and Sotalol

Amiodarone has a strong anti-arrhythmic effect thanks to its multiple mechanisms beyond acting as a class III drug, with blocking capacity of Na^+ and Ca channels++, and beta-blocking action reducing the dispersion of the ventricular action potential. Due to its modest negative inotropic effect, amiodarone is the most common and widely used drug in the treatment of electrical storm, especially in patients with structural heart disease. The efficacy of amiodarone in the treatment of electrical storm has been demonstrated in ad hoc clinical trials [10, 11].

The OPTIC study randomised a population of defibrillator patients with beta-blocker therapy vs. beta-blockers in combination with amiodarone vs. sotalol. The incidence of implantable cardioverter defibrillator (ICD) shocks was significantly lower in patients treated with the amiodarone–beta-blocker combination than in patients treated with beta-blockers alone [12]. Sotalol demonstrated a reduction in recurrences of ventricular arrhythmias compared to beta-blockers, but this difference was not statistically significant. In the context of out-of-hospital cardiac arrest, amiodarone, as well as lidocaine, was superior to placebo in improving survival to hospital admission, but neither amiodarone nor lidocaine was effective in improving survival to hospital discharge [13].

Lidocaine, Mexiletine, Procainamide and Quinidine

Sodium channel blockers are used in the treatment of electrical storm with uncertain results. Lidocaine blocks the rapid sodium current by a voltage- and use-dependent mechanism (it binds to the channel, blocking it during depolarisation and dissociating from it during electrical diastole); given the increased binding of the drug to the Na channel^{+}, it may be predominantly useful in the context of an electrical storm precipitated by acute myocardial ischaemia. It has been less effective in the treatment of patients with chronic ischaemic heart disease [14]. Mexiletine, when used in addition to amiodarone, has been shown to be effective in reducing the incidence of ICD interventions although its use tended to increase mortality in treated patients [15].

For their low negative inotropic effect, lidocaine and mexiletine can be safely used in patients with structural heart disease and in patients with chronic heart failure.

Procainamide, which similarly acts by blocking the rapid sodium current, has a stronger negative inotropic effect and, in patients with heart failure and advanced ventricular dysfunction, must be used with extreme caution. In patients with stable ventricular tachycardia (VT), procainamide has been shown to be more effective and safer than amiodarone [16].

Quinidine, beside blocking the fast Na^{+} current, is a blocker of the potassium currents Ikr and Ito. The particular action on Ito—whose alteration is at the basis of the dispersion of repolarisation in Brugada syndrome—accounts for the efficacy of this drug in reducing the incidence of malignant arrhythmias in channelopathies such as Brugada syndrome, early repolarisation syndrome, idiopathic ventricular fibrillation (VF) and short QT syndrome [17].

Quinidine has a modest negative inotropic effect and can therefore be considered in the treatment of patients with structural heart disease. A recent study by Li DL et al. demonstrated a moderate efficacy of quinidine, mostly in combination with other antiarrhythmic drugs, in the treatment of recurrent ventricular arrhythmias in patients with structural heart disease [18].

Isoproterenol

In some cases of marked bradycardia, VTs may also be triggered in the form of an electrical storm. The prevalent mechanism is torsade de pointes due to early afterdepolarisations triggered by bradycardia and/or by acquired QT prolongation. In such situations, pharmacological treatment of the electrical storm consists in the prompt suppression of the causes of bradycardia, such as electrolyte imbalance and drug overdose. In some cases, the administration of drugs with positive chronotropic effect—as isoproterenol—may be necessary. The use of isoproterenol in electrical storm is specifically indicated in Brugada syndrome, where recurrent episodes of VF are often favoured by vagal hypertone [19].

Deep Sedation

Hyperactivation of the sympathetic nervous system plays a key role in the onset and maintenance of electrical storm. There are various levels of cardiac autonomic nervous control: central (diencephalon and indirectly from the cortex), trunk, medullary, thoracic and cardio-cardiac. This dense multilevel control network, starting from the cortex, is the rationale for the use of deep sedation. Deep sedation has been shown to be effective in interrupting the vicious cycle that leads to nervous system activation and thus to the perpetuation of arrhythmic episodes. In a study by Bundgaard et al., on 15 patients with recurrent VT/FV electrical storm, deep sedation with propofol infusion resolved the electrical storm in 80% of the cases [20].

In a larger study by Martins et al., on 116 patients with electrical storm, deep sedation with midazolam and propofol suppressed arrhythmias within 15 min in about 50% of patients.

The good response to sedation in terms of arrhythmia suppression was associated with a significant reduction in in-hospital mortality [21]. The most widely used sedative drug for anti-arrhythmic purposes is propofol. This drug, in addition to its main hypnotic and sympatholytic action, can specifically act on ion channels in cardiomyocytes and cells of the cardiac conduction system. This interaction accounts for its anti-arrhythmic effect, as well as for some possible pro-arrhythmic risks [22].

Non-pharmacological Treatment

ICD Reprogramming

Implantable defibrillators (ICDs) have positively influenced survival in patients at increased risk of ventricular arrhythmias, with robust data supporting their superiority over antiarrhythmic drugs in both primary and secondary prevention. However, ICDs do not prevent ventricular arrhythmias. In ICD patients, the clinical presentation of the electrical storm is often characterised by multiple defibrillator interventions with ATP and shocks. These electrical therapies, albeit lifesaving, can represent severe distress for the patient, cause a further activation of the sympathetic system and favour the maintenance and recurrence of arrhythmias.

In their study of 2008, Poole et al. highlighted the association of ICD shocks and increased risk of mortality [23]; for this reason, in case of monomorphic and haemodynamically tolerated ventricular arrhythmias, it is suggested to switch off the ICD and to perform manual anti-tachycardia pacing. In ICD or biventricular pacemaker patients—with a possible pro-arrhythmic effect of left epicardial pacing—the pacing function can be switched off pending consideration of further therapeutic options [24]. In bradycardia-induced electrical storms, or in case of ventricular ectopic beats with a short-long-short cycle coupling phenomenon, it is possible to increase the lower pacing rate of the pacemaker/defibrillator.

Neuromodulation

Neuromodulation aims at reducing the activation of the sympathetic nervous system, which plays a role in the genesis and perpetuation of arrhythmias.

Thoracic epidural anaesthesia consists in the injection of a local anaesthetic into the epidural space of the thoracic ganglia; it can be performed at the patient's bedside or under fluoroscopic control, and it is effective in reducing electrical storm recurrences [25].

The *percutaneous left stellate ganglion block* technique is simpler, with a faster learning curve and more user-friendly, therefore easier to include in the treatment of electrical storm and in therapeutic flowcharts. The technique consists in injecting an anaesthetic at the level of the left stellate ganglion and can be performed at the patient's bedside with an anatomical approach or under ultrasound guidance. Several studies have confirmed its effectiveness in the treatment of electrical storms [26, 27].

Renal denervation consists in delivering radiofrequency inside the renal arteries with the aim of interfering with the sympathetic ganglia close to the renal arteries. This technique, originally developed for the treatment of resistant arterial hypertension, has proved effective in the treatment of refractory ventricular arrhythmias and electrical storm as well [28]. *Cardiac sympathetic denervation* is a surgical option, not suitable for the acute treatment of electrical storm but reasonable for the treatment of patients at risk of recurrences. In 2021, Dusi et al. described its application and positive outcomes in the treatment of channelopathy patients (long QT syndrome, catecholaminergic ventricular tachycardia) and in the treatment of ventricular arrhythmias refractory to traditional therapies [29]. More recently, the surgical technique of *thoracoscopic removal of the stellate ganglion* together with the first four thoracic ganglia has also been used in patients with structural heart disease and relapsing tachycardia. In this context, bilateral denervation proved to be more effective than the left mono-lateral technique alone; advanced heart failure and slow VT were significant predictors of procedural failure [30].

In our experience of patients with structural heart disease (¾ presenting with electrical storm), thoracoscopic bilateral cardiac denervation significantly reduced the incidence of both overall ventricular arrhythmias and electrical storm recurrences without a negative impact on cardiac performance [31]. Noteworthy, both the latest European guidelines on the treatment of ventricular arrhythmias and the recent consensus statement of European Heart Rhythm Association on the treatment of electrical storm highlight the importance of considering cardiac neuromodulation for both the acute treatment (i.e. stellate ganglion block) and for the prevention of the recurrences (i.e. cardiac denervation) of ventricular arrhythmias and electrical storm [32, 33].

Transcatheter Ablation

To date, transcatheter ablation has proved to be the most effective technique for the prevention of ventricular arrhythmic recurrences in the medium term. In few cases, ablation can be considered for the emergency management of electrical storm, but more often, it should be performed after patient stabilisation. Transcatheter ablation was initially considered as therapeutic option only in cases of stable monomorphic VT, where ventricular mapping during tachycardia was feasible, or in the few cases of evident repetitive extrasystolic beats that could trigger VT [34, 35]. More recently, thanks to new electro-anatomical mapping and substrate ablation techniques, the procedure could be extended to patients with haemodynamically poorly tolerated ventricular arrhythmias and/or with multiple forms of tachycardia [36, 37]. The effectiveness of transcatheter ablation has resulted in a significant improvement in prognosis in patients with electrical storm [38, 39]. It deserves to be emphasised that catheter ablation is a class I indication in patients with electrical storm and should be considered complementary rather than alternative to neuromodulation in most of the cases (Fig. 2.2) [32, 40].

Extracorporeal Circulation

In case of failure or impracticability of the treatments described above, the use of *extracorporeal circulation* (ECMO) may be considered as a bridge to other treatments. ECMO improves myocardial perfusion, reduces ventricular tele-diastolic

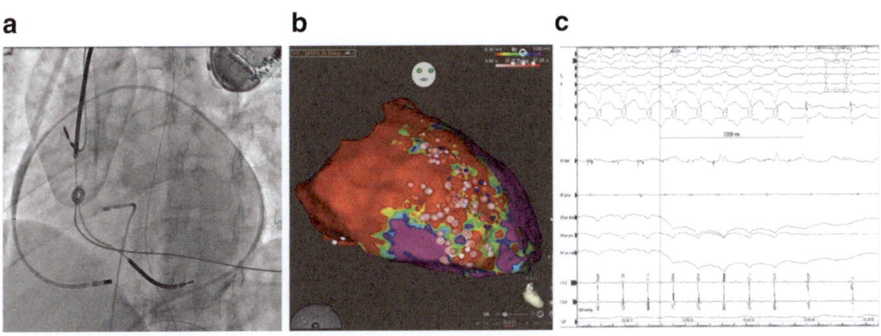

Fig. 2.2 Epicardial mapping and ablation in a patient with arrhythmogenic right ventricular heart disease and electrical storm. Panel **(a):** radioscopic image of the ablation catheter in the pericardial space. Panel (**b**): epicardial map of the right ventricle seen in a right oblique projection (red, scar areas with low-amplitude signal; red and pink dots, sites of delivery of radiofrequency for the treatment of tachycardia). Panel (**c**): interruption of one of the forms of tachycardia during radiofrequency delivery

pressure, may reduce sympathetic activation and allows the use of drugs with negative inotropic action. All these effects may contribute to restoring sinus rhythm, but the few studies available have also shown that more than half patients treated died during the therapy [41, 42]. The clinical presentation of alternating sinus rhythm and ventricular arrhythmias, when compared to the presence of refractory ventricular arrhythmias, proved to be a significant predictor of short-term survival. In 15% of patients, transcatheter ablation could be safely performed during ECMO therapy to treat the underlying causes of the electrical storm.

Radiotherapy of Arrhythmias

A new treatment of ventricular arrhythmias has been recently introduced in case of refractoriness to conventional therapies or when, owing to contraindications or excessive clinical instability, transcatheter ablation is discouraged. *Stereotactic ablation with radiotherapy* consists in delivering radiations to the area of the heart responsible for arrhythmias. Both Cuculich et al. in 2017 and Robinson et al. in 2019 reported encouraging results with a significant reduction in recurrences of ventricular arrhythmias and a good safety profile [43, 44]. In their study of 2020, Lloyd et al. observed a reduction of about 70% in episodes of ventricular arrhythmias after treatment with stereotactic radiotherapy in patients with ES [45]. To date, almost all clinical cases have been treated with a single fraction of 25Gy. In our facility, the first radiotherapy treatment with charged particles (protons) was carried out in a patient with ES that was refractory to drug therapy and to transcatheter ablation. Ventricular arrhythmias, frequent before radiotherapy, were suppressed almost immediately after treatment, and no recurrences were observed during the first 3 months of follow-up [46]. Radiotherapy for the treatment of arrhythmias represents a new promising noninvasive option, but its efficacy and safety need still further confirmation.

References

1. Elsokkari I, Tsuji Y, Sapp JL, Nattel S. Recent insights into mechanisms and clinical approaches to electrical storm. Can J Cardiol. 2021:S0828-282X(21)00969-7.
2. Exner DV, Pinski SL, Wyse DG, et al. Electrical storm presages nonsudden death: the antiarrhythmics versus implantable defibrillators (AVID) trial. Circulation. 2001;103:2066–71.
3. Guerra F, Shkoza M, Scappini L, Flori M, Capucci A. Role of electrical storm as a mortality and morbidity risk factor and its clinical predictors: a meta-analysis. Europace. 2013;16(3):347–53.
4. Elsokkari I, Parkash R, Tang A, et al. Mortality risk increases with clustered ventricular arrhythmias in patients with implantable cardioverter-defibrillators. JACC Clin Electrophysiol. 2020;6(3):327–37.
5. Hohnloser SH, Al-Khalidi HR, Pratt CM, et al. Electrical storm in patients with an implantable defibrillator: incidence, features, and preventive therapy: insights from a randomized trial. Eur Heart J. 2006;27(24):3027–32.
6. Guerra F, Bonelli P, Flori M, et al. Temporal trends and temperature-related incidence of electrical storm: the TEMPEST study (temperature-related incidence of electrical storm.). Circ Arrhythm Electrophysiol. 2017;10(3):e004634.

7. Nademanee K, Taylor R, Bailey WE, Rieders DE, Kosar EM. Treating electrical storm: sympathetic blockade versus advanced cardiac life support-guided therapy. Circulation. 2000;102(7):742–7.
8. Chatzidou S, Kontogiannis C, Tsilimigras DI, et al. Propranolol versus metoprolol for treatment of electrical storm in patients with implantable cardioverter-defibrillator. J Am Coll Cardiol. 2018;71(17):1897–906.
9. Miwa Y, Ikeda T, Mera H, Miyakoshi M, Hoshida K, Yanagisawa R, Ishiguro H, Tsukada T, Abe A, Yusu S, Yoshino H. Effects of landiolol, an ultra-short-acting beta1-selective blocker, on electrical storm refractory to class III antiarrhythmic drugs. Circ J. 2010;74(5):856–63.
10. Scheinman MM, Levine JH, Cannom DS, et al. Dose-ranging study of intravenous amiodarone in patients with life-threatening ventricular tachyarrhythmias. Circulation. 1995;92(11):3264–72.
11. Levine JH, Massumi A, Scheinman MM, et al. Intravenous amiodarone for recurrent sustained hypotensive ventricular tachyarrhythmias. J Am Coll Cardiol. 1996;27(1):67–75.
12. Connolly SJ, Dorian P, Roberts RS, et al. Comparison of β-blockers, amiodarone plus β-blockers, or sotalol for prevention of shocks from implantable cardioverter defibrillators: the OPTIC study: a randomised trial. JAMA. 2006;295(2):165–71.
13. Sanfilippo F, Corredor C, Santonocito C, et al. Amiodarone or lidocaine for cardiac arrest: a systematic review and meta-analysis. Resuscitation. 2016;107:31–7.
14. Nasir N Jr, Taylor A, Doyle TK, Pacifico A. Evaluation of intravenous lidocaine for the termination of sustained monomorphic ventricular tachycardia in patients with coronary artery disease with or without healed myocardial infarction. Am J Cardiol. 1994;74(12):1183–6.
15. Gao D, Van Herendael H, Alshengeiti L, et al. Mexiletine as an adjunctive therapy to amiodarone reduces the frequency of ventricular tachyarrhythmia events in patients with an implantable defibrillator. J Cardiovasc Pharmacol. 2013;62(2):199–204.
16. Ortiz M, Martin A, Arribas F, Coll-Vinent B, Del Arco C, Peinado R, et al. Randomized comparison of intravenous procainamide vs: intravenous amiodarone for the acute treatment of tolerated wide QRS tachycardia: the PROCAMIO study. Eur Heart J. 2017;38:1329–35.
17. Anguera I, Garcia-Alberola A, Dallaglio P, et al. Shock reduction with long-term quinidine in patients with Brugada syndrome and malignant ventricular arrhythmia episodes. J Am Coll Cardiol. 2016;67:1653–4.
18. Li DL, Cox ZL, Richardson TD, Kanagasundram AN, Saavedra PJ, Shen ST, Montgomery JA, Murray KT, Roden DM, Stevenson WG. Quinidine in the Management of Recurrent Ventricular Arrhythmias: a reappraisal. JACC Clin Electrophysiol. 2021;7(10):1254–63.
19. Ohgo T, Okamura H, Noda T, Satomi K, Suyama K, Kurita T, Aihara N, Kamakura S, Ohe T, Shimizu W. Acute and chronic management in patients with Brugada syndrome associated with electrical storm of ventricular fibrillation. Heart Rhythm. 2007;4(6):695–700.
20. Bundgaard JS, Jacobsen PK, Grand J, et al. Deep sedation as temporary bridge to definitive treatment of ventricular arrhythmia storm. Eur Heart J Acute Cardiovasc Care. 2020:2048872620903453.
21. Martins RP, Urien J-M, Barbarot N, et al. Effectiveness of deep sedation for patients with intractable electrical storm refractory to antiarrhythmic drugs. Circulation. 2020;142(16):1599–601.
22. Liu Q, Kong AL, Chen R, Qian C, Liu SW, Sun BG, Wang LX, Song LS, Hong J. Propofol and arrhythmias: two sides of the coin. Acta Pharmacol Sin. 2011;32(6):817–23.
23. Poole JE, Johnson GW, Hellkamp AS, et al. Prognostic importance of defibrillator shocks in patients with heart failure. N Engl J Med. 2008;359(10):1009–17.
24. Roque C, Trevisi N, Silberbauer J, Oloriz T, Mizuno H, Baratto F, et al. Electrical storm induced by cardiac resynchronization therapy is determined by pacing on epicardial scar and can be successfully managed by catheter ablation. Circ Arrhythm Electrophysiol. 2014;7:1064–9.
25. Do DH, Bradfield J, Ajijola OA, et al. Thoracic epidural anaesthesia can be effective for the short-term management of ventricular tachycardia storm. J Am Heart Assoc. 2017;6(11):e007080.
26. Meng L, Tseng C-H, Shivkumar K, Ajijola O. Efficacy of stellate ganglion blockade in managing electrical storm: a systematic review. JACC. 2017;3(9):942–9.

27. Savastano S, Dusi V, Baldi E, Rordorf R, Sanzo A, Camporotondo R, Fracchia R, Compagnoni S, Frigerio L, Oltrona Visconti L, De Ferrari GM. Anatomical-based percutaneous left stellate ganglion block in patients with drug-refractory electrical storm and structural heart disease: a single-centre case series. Europace. 2021;23(4):581–6.
28. Hawson J, Harmer JA, Cowan M, Virk S, Campbell T, Bennett RG, Anderson RD, Kalman J, Lee G, Kumar S. Renal denervation for the management of refractory ventricular arrhythmias: a systematic review. JACC Clin Electrophysiol. 2021;7(1):100–8.
29. Dusi V, Pugliese L, De Ferrari GM, et al. Left cardiac sympathetic denervation for long QT syndrome: 50 years' experience provides guidance for management. JACC Clin Eelectrophysiol. 2022;8(3):281–94.
30. Vaseghi M, Barwad P, Corrales FJM, et al. Cardiac sympathetic denervation for refractory ventricular arrhythmias. J Am Coll Cardiol. 2017;69(25):3070–80.
31. V Dusi, M Ruffinazzi, L Pugliese, F Guerrera, A Vicentini, S Savastano, , A Greco, R Camporotondo, S Frea, A Vairo, M Imazio, M Tritto, C Raineri, R Rordorf, GM De Ferrari. Impact of cardiac sympathetic denervation on electrical storms in patients with cardiomyopathies. Europace 2023 25 Supplement 1, i 519.
32. 2022 ESC Guidelines for the management of patients with ventricular arrhythmias and the prevention of sudden cardiac death. Eur Heart J 2022;43(40):3997–4126.
33. Lenarczyk R, Zeppenfeld K, Tfelt-Hansen J, Heinzel FR, Deneke T, Ene E, Meyer C, Wilde A, Arbelo E, Jędrzejczyk-Patej E, Sabbag A, Stühlinger M, di Biase L, Vaseghi M, Ziv O, Bautista-Vargas WF, Kumar S, Namboodiri N, Henz BD, Montero-Cabezas J, Dagres N, Peichl P, Frontera A, Tzeis S, Merino JL, Soejima K, de Chillou C, Tung R, Eckardt L, Maury P, Hlivak P, Tereshchenko LG, Kojodjojo P, Atié J. Management of patients with an electrical storm or clustered ventricular arrhythmias: a clinical consensus statement of the European Heart Rhythm Association of the ESC-endorsed by the Asia-Pacific Heart Rhythm Society, Heart Rhythm Society, and Latin-American Heart Rhythm Society. Europace. 2024;26(4):euae049.
34. Bänsch D, Oyang F, Antz M, et al. Successful catheter ablation of electrical storm after myocardial infarction. Circulation. 2003;108(24):3011–6.
35. Krisai P, Duchateau J, Cheniti G, Takagi T, Kamakura T, Ramirez FD, Pambrun T, Derval N, Sacher F, Jaïs P, Haïssaguerre M, Hocini M. Radiofrequency catheter ablation of ventricular fibrillation. Heart Rhythm. 2021;18(11):2016–7.
36. Schreieck J, Zrenner B, Deisenhofer I, Schmitt C. Rescue ablation of electrical storm in patients with ischemic cardiomyopathy: a potential-guided ablation approach by modifying substrate of intractable, unmappable ventricular tachycardias. Heart Rhythm. 2005;2(1):10–4.
37. Di Biase L, Santangeli P, Burkhardt DJ, Bai R, Mohanty P, Carbucicchio C, et al. Endoepicardial homogenization of the scar versus limited substrate ablation for the treatment of electrical storms in patients with ischemic cardiomyopathy. J Am Coll Cardiol. 2012;60:132–41.
38. Carbucicchio C, Santamaria M, Trevisi N, et al. Catheter ablation for the treatment of electrical storm in patients with implantable cardioverter-defibrillators. Circulation. 2008;117(4):462–9.
39. Vergara P, Tung R, Vaseghi M, Brombin C, Frankel DS, Di Biase L, Nagashima K, Tedrow U, Tzou WS, Sauer WH, Mathuria N, Nakahara S, Vakil K, Tholakanahalli V, Bunch TJ, Weiss JP, Dickfeld T, Vunnam R, Lakireddy D, Burkhardt JD, Correra A, Santangeli P, Callans D, Natale A, Marchlinski F, Stevenson WG, Shivkumar K, Della BP. Successful ventricular tachycardia ablation in patients with electrical storm reduces recurrences and improves survival. Heart Rhythm. 2018;15(1):48–55.
40. Savastano S, Baldi E, Rordorf R. Percutaneous stellate ganglion block and catheter ablation: not enemies but allies in fighting electrical storm. Eur Heart J. 2024:ehae276. Online ahead of print
41. Le Pennec-Prigent S, Flecher E, Auffret V, et al. Effectiveness of extracorporeal life support for patients with cardiogenic shock due to intractable electrical storm. Crit Care Med. 2017;45(3):e281–e9.
42. Baudry G, Sonneville R, Waintraub X, et al. Extracorporeal membrane oxygenation to support life-threatening drug-refractory electrical storm. Crit Care Med. 2020;48(10):e856–e63.

43. Cuculich PS, Schill MR, Kashani R, et al. Noninvasive cardiac radiation for ablation of ventricular tachycardia. N Engl J Med. 2017;377(24):2325–36.
44. Robinson CG, Samson PP, Moore KM, et al. Phase I/II trial of electrophysiology guided noninvasive cardiac radioablation for ventricular tachycardia. Circulation. 2019;139(3):313–21.
45. Lloyd MS, Wight J, Schneider F, et al. Clinical experience of stereotactic body radiation for refractory ventricular tachycardia in advanced heart failure patients. Heart Rhythm. 2020;17(3):415–22.
46. Dusi V, Vitolo V, Frigerio L, Totaro R, Valentini A, Barcellini A, Mirandola A, Perego GB, Coccia M, Greco A, Ghio S, Valvo F, De Ferrari GM, Gnecchi M, Oltrona Visconti L, Rordorf R. First-in-man case of non-invasive proton radiotherapy for the treatment of refractory ventricular tachycardia in advanced heart failure. Eur J Heart Fail. 2021;23(1):195–6.

The Autonomic Nervous System and Ventricular Arrhythmias

3

Veronica Dusi and Gaetano Maria De Ferrari

Introduction

The heart is richly innervated by afferent (sensory) and efferent (or visceromotor) nerves, the latter divided into a sympathetic and a parasympathetic branch. Their activity is finely integrated within a complex series of peripheral and central feedback circuits that allow the autonomic control of cardiac function. The entire autonomic nervous system (ANS) aims at maintaining cardiac homeostasis in the face of internal and external perturbations, ensuring appropriate and timely responses to stimuli. However, in pathological conditions such as myocardial infarction/ischaemia and heart failure, autonomic reflexes can become detrimental and lead to life-threatening arrhythmias and progression of myocardial dysfunction. In this section, we will first discuss the anatomy and then the basic physiology and pathophysiology of cardiac ANS, focusing both on the role of ANS in the genesis of ventricular arrhythmias (VA) and on the rationale for cardiac sympathetic blockade interventions for antiarrhythmic purposes [1].

Functional Anatomy of the Cardiac Neuraxis

The cardiac neuraxis is divided into two systems: the intracardiac, or intrinsic cardiac nervous system (ICNS), and the extracardiac, or extrinsic system, both of which contain afferent and efferent fibres. The two efferent branches of the cardiac autonomic

(translated by Chiara Barbaglia)

V. Dusi · G. M. De Ferrari (✉)
Department of Medical Sciences, University of Turin, Turin, Italy

Division of Cardiology, Azienda Ospedaliero-Universitaria Città della Salute e della Scienza – Torino, Torino, Italy
e-mail: gaetanomaria.deferrari@unito.it

S. Savastano (ed.), *Percutaneous Stellate Ganglion Block for Electrical Storm*,
https://doi.org/10.1007/978-3-031-81762-5_3

nervous system, the sympathetic and the parasympathetic systems, share a common embryonic origin from the neural crest. Generally, afferent fibres, albeit improperly, are also defined as sympathetic or parasympathetic afferent fibres, depending on their anatomical course and on the kind of reflex responses that their stimulation elicits, attesting the close anatomo-functional correlation of these responses. The intrinsic cardiac nervous system (ICNS) consists of a network of interconnected ganglia and nerves located in multiple ganglionic plexuses (GPs) in the epicardial fat pads [2]. The extracardiac nervous system includes the mediastinal plexus, the cervico-thoracic ganglia, the nodose ganglia, the dorsal root ganglia (DRG), the spinal cord and the brainstem. The cardiac sympathetic ANS follows a typical course in most people, although variants can be observed. The efferent sympathetic preganglionic neurons have their soma located in the intermedio-lateral column [3] of the grey matter of the spinal cord and contract synapses with postganglionic neurons located in the last of the paravertebral cervical sympathetic ganglia and the first thoracic ganglia. The lowest cervical ganglion (C8) and the highest thoracic ganglion (T1) are generally fused bilaterally, forming the left and right stellate ganglia (also called the cervico-thoracic ganglia). In less than 3% of human sympathetic chains, the second thoracic ganglion (T2) is also fused, forming a trilobed stellate ganglion (C8-T1-T2). A substantial amount of postganglionic cardiac sympathetic fibres originates from the stellate ganglia. The rest is supplied mainly by the T2–T4 paravertebral ganglia, although some studies suggest a contribution also from the middle cervical ganglia [4] and, very modestly, also from T5 [5]. Axons from these ganglia reach the heart via the cardiopulmonary nerves. In addition, a small number of cardiac sympathetic postganglionic neurons is found in each of the main ganglia of the ICNS [6].

The soma of the efferent parasympathetic preganglionic neurons is mainly located in the ventral lateral region of the nucleus ambiguus, giving rise to the vagus nerve in the periphery. The vagus trunk is a mixed nerve, consisting of about 80% A∂ and C-type afferent fibres and about 20% B-type efferent fibres. The cardiomotor fibres project onto the parasympathetic neurons of the ICNS ganglia. The cardiac vagal branches, together with the cardiopulmonary (sympathetic) nerves, form the mediastinal plexus. Finally, the nerve bodies of the cardiac afferent neurons are located in the nodose ganglia, in the dorsal root ganglia of the spinal modulus from C7 to T4 [7], as well as in the intrinsic cardiac ganglia of the ICNS [8], thus providing the anatomical basis for cardiac neuronal control at multiple levels (intracardiac, spinal and central).

The ICNS is also called the 'little brain' of the heart [9], as it is the first independent station of the cardiac ANS. The ICNS enables local reflex control, beat by beat, of all cardiac functions and responses, as well as integration and coordination with the higher centres for medium- and long-term reflexes. This is possible due to the presence within it of sensory afferent neurons, efferent motor neurons, local circuit neurons (neurons that project axons only to adjacent neurons) and interneurons (neurons that project axons to other ganglia). Most efferent neurons in the ICNS are cholinergic and respond to preganglionic control of the efferent fibres of the vagus nerve. The cholinergic and adrenergic neurons contained in each atrial and ventricular ganglionic plexus preferentially control different regions of the heart, albeit with a high degree of overlapping [10]. In humans, the highest density of ICNS neurons

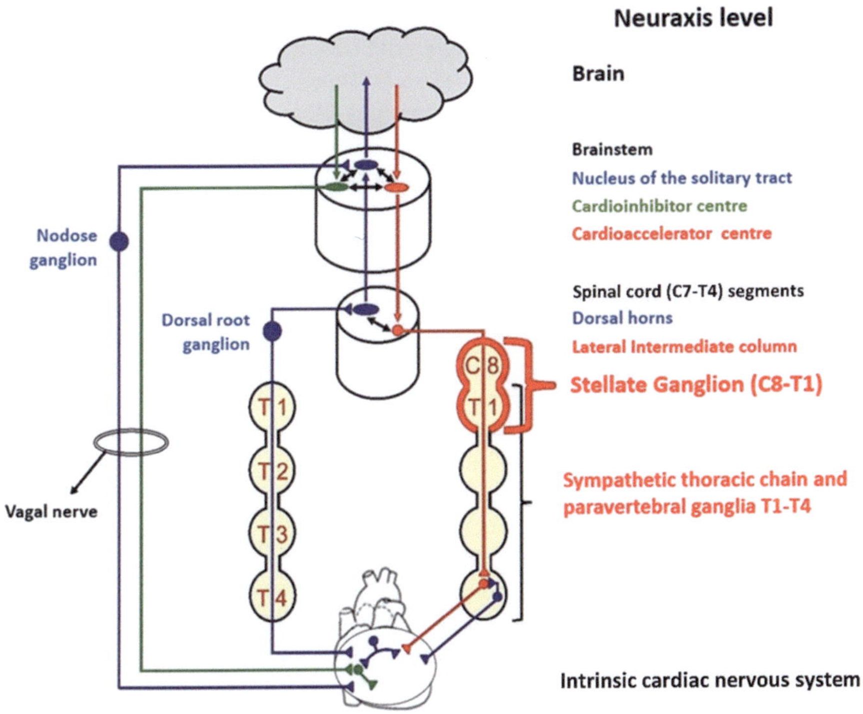

Fig. 3.1 Organisation of the cardiac nervous system in humans. Blue: afferent nervous system with its ganglia: nodose ganglia and dorsal root ganglia (DRG) from C7 to T4. Green: parasympathetic efferent nervous system. Red: sympathetic efferent nervous system. All afferent and efferent structures outside the central nervous system are bilateral, although most are represented as unilateral for simplicity. Cardiac afferent fibres spreading through the paravertebral sympathetic ganglia (usually referred to as cardiac sympathetic afferent fibres) reach the DRGs directly without contracting synapses. These fibres mediate cardiac sympathetic spinal reflexes that significantly increase efferent sympathetic activity directed to the heart. Left cardiac sympathetic denervation (LCSD) consists in the removal of the left thoracic sympathetic chain and paravertebral ganglia from T1 to T4. Since the ipsilateral DRGs are spared by LCSD, left afferent reinnervation from the DRGs to the heart might be possible with time. The left efferent sympathetic system from T1 to T4 is instead interrupted at a preganglionic level; therefore, no ipsilateral efferent sympathetic reinnervation is possible after LCSD. (Modified from Dusi V [71])

lies on the posterior surface of the atria. Figure 3.1 summarises the organisation of the cardiac nervous system in humans.

Historical Perspective

In 1899, Francois-Frank [11] was the first to suggest that removal of the cervicothoracic sympathetic ganglia could prevent episodes of angina pectoris. The first operation was performed in 1916 by Jonnesco [12]: the surgeon removed the left stellate ganglion (LSG) in a patient suffering from recurrent angina associated with cardiac arrhythmias, with effective and lasting suppression of both conditions. This pioneering intervention was later strongly criticised due to the potentially harmful effects of depriving patients of the alarm signal represented by pain. Furthermore, the consequences of left stellectomy on coronary blood flow were still unclear. In 1929, Leriche and Fontaine [13] demonstrated that the sympathetic nerves exerted a vasoconstrictor effect on the coronary arteries and not a vasodilator effect, as previously thought. Subsequently, numerous clinical studies were conducted in both Europe and the USA, confirming that left stellectomy could prevent anginal attacks [14] and improve exercise tolerance [15] in patients with ischaemic heart disease. Regarding the optimal extent of the procedure, cervico-thoracic denervation (removal of the stellate ganglion and thoracic ganglia from T2 to T4) proved to be the most effective. Finally, since the 1960s, despite its efficacy, left cardiac sympathetic denervation (LCSD, consisting of removal of the thoracic sympathetic ganglia from T1 to T4) for antianginal purposes was progressively abandoned due to the advent of coronary artery bypass and later on β-blockers [16].

With the exception of a few anecdotal clinical cases [17, 18], the antiarrhythmic potential use of cardiac sympathetic denervation (LCSD) in humans remained largely unexplored until the 1970s. In 1971, Moss and McDonald [19] first used LCSD in a patient with congenital long QT syndrome (LQTS) and recurrent syncopal episodes. The rationale was based on a canine study by Yanowiz [20] in 1966 showing a consistent prolongation of the QT interval after both right stellate gangliectomy and LSG stimulation. The patient underwent removal of the left sympathetic ganglia from C7 to T2, including the entire LSG. In addition to the suppression of ventricular arrhythmias, a persistent reduction of the QT interval was also noted. Subsequently, other groups attempted to reproduce the beneficial effects of LCSD on the QT interval through reversible percutaneous blockade of the LSG, with mixed results [21]. Importantly, at that time, the onset of Horner's syndrome was considered a good indicator of effective cardiac nerve block. On the contrary, as pointed out as early as 1975 [22], Horner's syndrome simply indicates effective blockade of the sympathetic fibres that travel in the upper part of the stellate ganglion and innervate the eye. It does not necessarily indicate blockage of the sympathetic fibres that reach the heart, as also recently confirmed by larger human studies clearly showing that the antiarrhythmic efficacy of percutaneous LSG block was not associated with the onset of Horner's syndrome [23]. Furthermore, unlike in dogs and in cats, in humans, cardiac sympathetic innervation is not entirely provided by the stellate ganglia.

A better understanding of the rationale for LCSD in LQTS originated from the study by PJ Schwartz's group. Schwartz started from the clinical observation that in his first patient with LQTS, sympathetic activation (represented by physical or emotional stress conditions) led to the onset of electrocardiographic macroscopic T-wave alternance, a pattern that he was able to reproduce in cats (both QT interval lengthening and alternation) by electrical stimulation of the LSG [24]. On this basis, the young patient was treated with LCSD, remaining asymptomatic for over 40 years, and sympathetic imbalance with left-sided dominance was proposed as the pathophysiological mechanism of LQTS [25]. This concept stimulated a wide range of experimental studies aimed at investigating the consequences of unilateral (right or left) cardiac sympathetic denervation on the heart [26–30].

Antiarrhythmic Rationale and Mechanisms of Action of Cardiac Sympathetic Blockade

Antiadrenergic Effects

In 1976, Schwartz et al. demonstrated in anaesthetised dogs [26] that ventricular arrhythmias associated with acute myocardial ischaemia were increased by right stellate ganglion block and decreased by LSG block. The protective effect of left stellectomy was subsequently confirmed in a conscious canine model [27], which is still considered one of the most clinically relevant experimental models of SCD (dogs with a previous anterior myocardial infarction exposed to a short acute coronary occlusion during treadmill exercise). The antagonism of the excitatory sympathetic reflex induced by acute myocardial ischaemia [28] and the quantitative dominance, at the level of the left ventricle, of the left-sided sympathetic nerves over the right [29] were the first antiarrhythmic mechanisms proposed for protection associated with blockade or removal of the LSG. It was subsequently shown that the threshold of ventricular fibrillation, a reliable and quantitative indicator of cardiac electrical stability, was much higher after left stellectomy [30]. These animal data provide a strong rationale for cardiac sympathetic blockade interventions, both temporary and definitive, that goes well beyond LQTS [31] and myocardial ischaemia-related arrhythmias [32] and could potentially extend to any cardiac condition of increased susceptibility to the development of malignant ventricular arrhythmias. It is believed that the most important mechanism involved in the anti-arrhythmic protection is the marked decrease in norepinephrine (NE) released in the left ventricle during sympathetic nerve activation. Indeed, it must be taken into account that NE release from nerve endings is an extremely inhomogeneous phenomenon in time and space [33, 34]: as proof of this, it has been shown that sympathetic nerve activation, but not circulating NE, modulates the T-peak to T-end interval (an ECG marker of repolarisation dispersion) by increasing the overall spatial dispersion of repolarisation [35, 36]. In turn, the spatial dispersion of ventricular repolarisation is a very well-established pro-arrhythmic marker, both for anatomical re-entry arrhythmias [37] and for functional re-entry arrhythmias such as polymorphic ventricular tachycardia and VF [38]. Temporal dispersion of ventricular repolarisation is also important and, together with spatial dispersion, can lead to T-wave alternance, an electrocardiographic marker of electrical instability, in case of both macroscopic and microscopic alternace [39]. Finally, it has also been shown that, while there is a marginal effect of increasing conduction velocity in healthy hearts [40], in case of myocardial scar, sympathetic activation modulates conduction velocity in the peri-infarct region in a very heterogeneous space, resulting in a significant delay of local activation times. This is a further mechanism linking sympathetic activation to an enhanced risk of re-entry arrhythmias [41]. Moreover, NE, like epinephrine, besides acting on the arrhythmic substrate, also modulates the trigger by increasing both automatism in myocardial conduction cells (at the atrial and ventricular level) [42] and triggered activity in the form of both early (EAD) [43] and late (DAD) [44, 45] afterdepolarisation. Additional neurotransmitters released by sympathetic efferent fibers in the setting of high level activation, such as neuropeptide Y (NPY), are also gaining increasing attention due to their proarrhythmic potential [46]. Finally, cardiac sympathetic block also has anti α-adrenergic effects, which, as opposed to pure anti β-adrenergic effects, have a vasodilating effect on the coronary circulation. Indeed, LCSD increases myocardial reactive hyperaemia, an index of the coronaries' ability to dilate [47]. In addition to providing the basis for the antianginal effect, this contributes to the anti-arrhythmic efficacy [48].

Vagotonic Effect

Animal studies have clearly shown that LCSD is accompanied by a reflex increase in cardiac parasympathetic (vagal) efferent activity [49]. Indeed, LCSD interrupts most centrally projected cardiac sympathetic afferents, which have an inhibitory effect on cardiac vagal output. In turn, experimental [50, 51] and clinical data [52, 53] have shown that the reduction of both tonic and phasic (reflex) cardiac vagal activity may trigger malignant ventricular arrhythmias; conversely, such arrhythmias can be counteracted in animals by electrical stimulation of the vagus nerve [54] or pharmacological activation [55]. So far, direct experience with electrical vagus nerve stimulation for cardiac conditions in humans is limited to patients with heart failure [56–58]. The vagotonic effect of LCSD is particularly relevant from an anti-arrhythmic point of view in conditions characterised by a chronic and progressive increase in sympathetic tone and a parallel decrease in central parasympathetic drive, such as myocardial infarction (MI) and reperfusion [59] and heart failure [60]. Also, due to the complexity of sympathetic-parasympathetic interactions, a vagotonic effect has also the potential to enhance cardiac contractility [61]. Some of these concepts are at the basis of an ongoing clinical trial examining the potential benefits associated with LCSD in patients with advanced heart failure [62].

Further Effects of Cardiac Sympathetic Blockade on the Heart

Catecholamines, in addition to their arrhythmogenic potential, physiologically modulate almost all cardiac functions, including inotropism, chronotropism, dromotropism, batmotropism, and lusitropism. Therefore, prior to systematically proposing the clinical use of cardiac sympathetic blockade in humans, either transiently or permanently (LCSD), several experimental studies were conducted to rule out potential harmful effects on the heart. In conscious dogs with a stabilised myocardial infarction who performed a submaximal exercise test, left ventricular contractility (assessed by dP/dt max) was not affected by left stellectomy [47]. Furthermore, left stellectomy did not reduce resting heart rate (HR) or chronotropic competence during exercise. In contrast, the observed increase in HR during exercise was slightly (6%) greater than at baseline. The explanation given for this apparently paradoxical phenomenon was that it could be related to a reflex increase in the activity of the contralateral right stellate ganglion. Indeed, due to the asymmetric distribution of the cardiac sympathetic nerves, the sinus node is under predominant right sympathetic control [5]. In the same animal model [47] the maximum increase in HR during exercise was, respectively, 19% and 26% lower than at baseline (innervation intact) after bilateral stellectomy and after right-only stellectomy. Finally, although the study did not provide specific data on atrioventricular conduction, the maximum mean HR reached (about 250 bpm) during exercise after left stellectomy leads to the supposition that there is no significant impact of left stellectomy on dromotropism during sinus rhythm and under physiological conditions of sympathetic activation. This result was in full agreement with previous studies showing that sympathetic innervation of the atria and atrioventricular node was provided by both the right and left sympathetic chains [63]. As proof of this, recent data from patients with paroxysmal atrial fibrillation (AF) show equivalent electrophysiological effects of temporary blockade of the right or left stellate ganglion with lidocaine on the common atrial myocardium: unilateral blockade, regardless of the side of application, slightly prolongs the effective atrial refractory period and consistently reduces the inducibility of AF and the duration of AF episodes [64]. Also, recent data from patients with cardiomyopathy undergoing bilateral cardiac sympathetic denervation for antiarrhythmic purposes indicate a mild but significant effect on chronotropism, with no discernible impact on dromotropism at rest [69].

Finally, a further concern was that LCSD could lead to post denervation supersensitivity, a pro-arrhythmic condition characterised by an increased left ventricular sensitivity to catecholamines after complete denervation. In theory, this possibility seemed unlikely, since the right-sided sympathetic nerves, preserved after LCSD, also contribute to the innervation of the left ventricle [66, 67]. Animal studies confirmed that catecholamine reserves in the myocardium were not completely depleted after LCSD [68, 69]. Furthermore, unilateral left stellectomy did not increase the incidence of ventricular arrhythmias in response to intravenous noradrenaline [70]. LCSD is a preganglionic efferent denervation; therefore, ipsilateral sympathetic efferent reinnervation is not possible, unlike what occurs following cardiac transplantation, where efferent sympathetic denervation is postganglionic (paravertebral sympathetic chains are intact) and reinnervation is therefore possible. On the contrary, similarly to the post-cardiac transplant condition, the afferent ganglionic stations located at the level of the posterior roots of the spinal nerves (DRGs) are unaffected by the intervention (postganglionic afferent denervation). It follows that, as opposed to the acute afferent sympathetic block, an afferent regenerative potential—though very difficult to study in vivo—may occur at least partially within years.

References

1. Dusi V, Zhu C, Ajijola OA. Neuromodulation approaches for cardiac arrhythmias: recent advances current cardiology reports. 2019;21(5). https://doi.org/10.1007/s11886-019-1120-1.
2. Armour JA, Murphy DA, Yuan BX, Mac Donald S, Hopkins DA. Gross and microscopic anatomy of the human intrinsic cardiac nervous system. Anat Rec. 1997;247:289–98.

3. Vincentz JW, Rubart M, Firulli AB. Ontogeny of cardiac sympathetic innervation and its implications for cardiac disease. Pediatr Cardiol. 2012;33:923–8. https://doi.org/10.1007/s00246-012-0248-1.
4. Irie T, Yamakawa K, Hamon D, Nakamura K, Shivkumar K, Vaseghi M. Cardiac sympathetic innervation via middle cervical and stellate ganglia and antiarrhythmic mechanism of bilateral stellectomy. Am J Physiol Heart Circ Physiol. 2017;312:H392–405. https://doi.org/10.1152/ajpheart.00644.2016.
5. Randall WC, Rohse WG. The augmentor action of the sympathetic cardiac nerves. Circ Res. 1956;4(4):470–5. https://doi.org/10.1161/01.res.4.470.
6. The intrinsic cardiac nervous system: from pathophysiology to therapeutic implications biology. 2024;13(2):105. https://doi.org/10.3390/biology13020105.
7. Andresen MC, Kuntz DL, Mendelowitz D. In: Armour JA, Ardell JL, editors. Central nervous system regulation of the heart. New York: Oxford University Press; 2004. p. 187–219.
8. Hopkins DA, Andrew AJ. Ganglionic distribution of afferent neurons innervating the canine heart and cardiopulmonary nerves. J Auton Nerv Syst. 1989;26:213–22.
9. Armour JA. Potential clinical relevance of the “little brain” on the mammalian heart. Exp Physiol. 2008;93:165–76. https://doi.org/10.1113/expphysiol.2007.041178.
10. Pauza DH, Skripka V, Pauziene N, Stropus R. Morphology, distribution, and variability of the epicardiac neural ganglionated subplexes in the human heart. Anat Rec. 2000;259:353–82.
11. Francois-Frank CA. Signification physiologique de la resection du sympathique dans la maladie de Basedow, l'epilepsie, l'idiotic et le glaucoma. Bull Acad Méd Paris. 1989;41:565–94.
12. Jonnesco T. Traitement chirurgical de l'angine de poitrine par la résection du sympathique cervico-thoracique [French]. Presse Méd. 1921;20:221–30.
13. Leriche R, Fontaine R. Rôle du ganglion étoile gauche dans le déterminisme de la crise de l'angine de poitrine [French]. C R Acad Sci. 1929;188:279–80.
14. Burnett CF, Evans JA. Follow-up report on resection of the anginal pathway in thirty-three patients. JAMA. 1956;162:709–12. https://doi.org/10.1001/jama.1956.02970250009003.
15. Cox WV. Influence of stellate ganglion block on angina pectoris and the post-exercise ECG. Am J Med. 1956;252:289–95.
16. Schwartz PJ. The rationale and the role of left stellectomy for the prevention of malignant arrhythmias. Ann N Y Acad Sci. 1984;427:199–221. https://doi.org/10.1111/j.1749-6632.1984.tb20785.x.
17. Estes EH, Izlar HR. Recurrent ventricular tachycardia: a case successfully treated by bilateral cardiac sympathectomy. Am J Med. 1961;31:493–7. https://doi.org/10.1016/0002-9343(61)90132-2.
18. Zipes DP, Festoff B, Schaal SF, Cox C, Sealy WC, Wallace AG. Treatment of ventricular arrhythmia by permanent atrial pacemaker and cardiac sympathectomy. Ann Intern Med. 1968;68:591–7. https://doi.org/10.7326/0003-4819-68-3-591.
19. Moss AJ, McDonald J. Unilateral cervicothoracic sympathetic ganglionectomy for the treatment of long QT interval syndrome. N Engl J Med. 1971;285:903–4. https://doi.org/10.1056/NEJM197110142851607.
20. Yanowitz F, Preston JB, Abildskov JA. Functional distribution of right and left stellate innervation to the ventricles: production of neurogenic electrocardiographic changes by unilateral alteration of sympathetic tone. Circ Res. 1966;18:416–28. https://doi.org/10.1161/01.RES.18.4.416.
21. Schwartz PJ. Cardiac sympathetic denervation to prevent life-threatening arrhythmias. Nat Rev Cardiol. 2014;11:346–53. https://doi.org/10.1038/nrcardio.2014.19.
22. Schwartz PJ, Periti M, Malliani A. The long QT syndrome. Am Heart J. 1975;89:378–90. https://doi.org/10.1016/0002-8703(75)90089-7.
23. Correction to: Electrical storm treatment by percutaneous stellate ganglion block: the STAR study. Eur. Heart J. 2024;45(39):4235. https://doi.org/10.1093/eurheartj/ehae631.
24. Schwartz PJ, Malliani A. Electrical alternation of the T wave: clinical and experimental evidence of its relationship with the sympathetic nervous system and with the long QT syndrome. Am Heart J. 1975;89:45–50. https://doi.org/10.1016/0002-8703(75)90008-3.

25. Schwartz PJ. Idiopathic long QT syndrome: progress and questions. Am Heart J. 1985;109:399–411. https://doi.org/10.1016/0002-8703(85)90626-X.
26. Schwartz PJ, Stone HL, Brown AM. Effects of unilateral stellate ganglion blockade on the arrhythmias associated with coronary occlusion. Am Heart J. 1976;92:589–99. https://doi.org/10.1016/S0002-8703(76)80078-6.
27. Schwartz PJ, Billman GE, Stone HL. Autonomic mechanisms in ventricular fibrillation induced by myocardial ischemia during exercise in dogs with healed myocardial infarction: an experimental preparation for sudden cardiac death. Circulation. 1984;69:790–800. https://doi.org/10.1161/01.CIR.69.4.790.
28. Schwartz PJ. Sympathetic imbalance and cardiac arrythmias. In: Randall WC, editor. Nervous control of cardiovascular function. New York, NY: Oxford: Oxford University Press; 1984. p. 225–52.
29. Malliani A, Schwartz PJ, Zanchetti A. A sympathetic reflex elicited by experimental coronary occlusion. Am J Phys. 1969;217:703–9. https://doi.org/10.1152/ajplegacy.1969.217.3.703.
30. Schwartz PJ, Snebold NG, Brown AM. Effects of unilateral cardiac sympathetic denervation on the ventricular fibrillation threshold. Am J Cardiol. 1976;37:1034–40. https://doi.org/10.1016/0002-9149(76)90420-3.
31. Left cardiac sympathetic denervation for long QT syndrome JACC: clinical electrophysiology. 2022;8(3):281–94. https://doi.org/10.1016/j.jacep.2021.09.002.
32. Physical inactivity is a risk factor for primary ventricular fibrillation. JACC. 2019;73(16):2117–8. https://doi.org/10.1016/j.jacc.2019.01.063.
33. Han J, Moe GK. Nonuniform recovery of excitability in ventricular muscle. Circ Res. 1964;14:44–60. https://doi.org/10.1161/01.RES.14.1.44.
34. Opthof T, Misier AR, Coronel R, Vermeulen JT, Verberne HJ, Frank RG, et al. Dispersion of refractoriness in canine ventricular myocardium. Effects of sympathetic stimulation. Circ Res. 1991;68:1204–15. https://doi.org/10.1161/01.RES.68.5.1204.
35. Ramirez RJ, Ajijola OA, Zhou W, Holmström B, Lüning H, Laks MM, et al. A new electrocardiographic marker for sympathetic nerve stimulation: modulation of repolarization by stimulation of stellate ganglia. J Electrocardiol. 2011;44:694–9. https://doi.org/10.1016/j.jelectrocard.2011.07.030.
36. Yagishita D, Chui RW, Yamakawa K, Rajendran PS, Ajijola OA, Nakamura K, et al. Sympathetic nerve stimulation, not circulating norepinephrine, modulates T-peak to T-end interval by increasing global dispersion of repolarization. Circ Arrhythm Electrophysiol. 2015;8:174–85. https://doi.org/10.1161/CIRCEP.114.002195.
37. Vaseghi M, Lux RL, Mahajan A, Shivkumar K. Sympathetic stimulation increases dispersion of repolarization in humans with myocardial infarction. Am J Physiol Heart Circ Physiol. 2012;302:H1838–H46. https://doi.org/10.1152/ajpheart.01106.2011.
38. Antzelevitch C. Role of spatial dispersion of repolarization in inherited and acquired sudden cardiac death syndromes. Am J Physiol Heart Circ Physiol. 2007;293:H2024–H38. https://doi.org/10.1152/ajpheart.00355.2007.
39. Nearing BD, Oesterle SN, Verrier RL. Quantification of ischaemia-induced vulnerability by precordial T-wave alternans analysis in dog and human. Cardiovasc Res. 1994;28:1440–9. https://doi.org/10.1093/cvr/28.9.1440.
40. Wallace AG, Sarnoff SJ. Effects of cardiac sympathetic nerve stimulation on conduction in the heart. Circ Res. 1964;14:86–92. https://doi.org/10.1161/01.res.14.1.86.
41. Ajijola OA, Lux RL, Khahera A, Kwon O, Aliotta E, Ennis DB, Fishbein MC, Ardell JL, Shivkumar K. Sympathetic modulation of electrical activation in normal and infarcted myocardium: implications for arrhythmogenesis. Am J Physiol Heart Circ Physiol. 2017;312(3):H608–21. https://doi.org/10.1152/ajpheart.00575.2016.
42. Zipes DP, Barber MJ, Takahashi N, Gilmour RF Jr. Influence of the autonomic nervous system on the genesis of cardiac arrhythmias. Pacing Clin Electrophysiol. 1983;6:1210–20. https://doi.org/10.1111/j.1540-8159.1983.tb04459.x.

43. Ben-David J, Zipes DP. Differential response to right and left ansae subclaviae stimulation of early afterdepolarizations and ventricular tachycardia induced by cesium in dogs. Circulation. 1988;78:1241–50. https://doi.org/10.1161/01.CIR.78.5.1241.
44. Charpentier F, Drouin E, Gauthier C, LeMarec H. Early after/depolarizations and triggered activity: mechanisms and autonomic regulation. Fundam Clin Pharmacol. 1993;7:39–49. https://doi.org/10.1111/j.1472-8206.1993.tb00216.x.
45. Priori SG, Mantica M, Schwartz PJ. Delayed after depolarisations elicited in vivo by left stellate ganglion stimulation. Circulation. 1988;78:178–85. https://doi.org/10.1161/01.CIR.78.1.178.
46. Dusi V, De Ferrari GM, Schwartz PJ. There are 100 ways by which the sympathetic nervous system can trigger life-threatening arrhythmias. Abstract Eur. Heart J. 2020;41(23):2180–2. https://doi.org/10.1093/eurheartj/ehz950.
47. Schwartz PJ, Stone HL. Effects of unilateral stellectomy upon cardiac performance during exercise in dogs. Circ Res. 1979;44:637–45. https://doi.org/10.1161/01.RES.44.5.637.
48. Schwartz PJ, Vanoli E, Zaza A, Zuanetti G. The effect of antiarrhythmic drugs on life-threatening arrhythmias induced by the interaction between acute myocardial ischemia and sympathetic hyperactivity. Am Heart J. 1985;109:937–48. https://doi.org/10.1016/0002-8703(85)90233-9.
49. Cerati D, Schwartz PJ. Single cardiac vagal fibers activity, acute myocardial ischemia, and risk for sudden death. Circ Res. 1991;69:1389–401. https://doi.org/10.1161/01.RES.69.5.1389.
50. Billman GE, Schwartz PJ, Stone HL. Baroreceptor reflex control of heart rate: a predictor of sudden cardiac death. Circulation. 1982;66:874–80. https://doi.org/10.1161/01.CIR.66.4.874.
51. Schwartz PJ, Vanoli E, Stramba-Badiale M, De Ferrari GM, Billman GE, Foreman RD. Autonomic mechanisms and sudden death: new insights from analysis of baroreceptor reflexes in conscious dogs with and without a myocardial infarction. Circulation. 1998;78:969–79. https://doi.org/10.1161/01.CIR.78.4.969.
52. Oak MT, Bigger JT Jr, Marcus FI, Mortara A, Schwartz PJ. Baroreflex sensitivity and heart-rate variability in prediction of total cardiac mortality after myocardial infarction. Lancet. 1998;351:478–84. https://doi.org/10.1016/S0140-6736(97)11144-8.
53. La Rovere MT, Pinna GD, Hohnloser SH, Marcus FI, Mortara A, Nohara R, et al. Baroreflex sensitivity and heart rate variability in the identification of patients at risk for life-threatening arrhythmias: implications for clinical trials. Circulation. 2001;103:2072–7. https://doi.org/10.1161/01.CIR.103.16.2072.
54. Vanoli E, De Ferrari GM, Stramba-Badiale M, Hull SS Jr, Foreman RD, Schwartz PJ. Vagal stimulation and prevention of sudden death in conscious dogs with a healed myocardial infarction. Circ Res. 1991;68:1471–81. https://doi.org/10.1161/01.RES.68.5.1471.
55. De Ferrari GM, Vanoli E, Curcuruto P, Tommasini G, Schwartz PJ. Prevention of life-threatening arrhythmias by pharmacologic stimulation of the muscarinic receptors with oxotremorine. Am Heart J. 1992;124:883–90. https://doi.org/10.1016/0002-8703(92)90968-2.
56. De Ferrari GM, Crijns HJ, Borggrefe M, Milasinovic G, Smid J, Zabel M, et al. Chronic vagus nerve stimulation: a new and promising therapeutic approach for chronic heart failure. Eur Heart J. 2011;32:847–55. https://doi.org/10.1093/eurheartj/ehq391.
57. Dusi V, De Ferrari GM. Vagal stimulation in heart failure. Herz. 2021;46(6):541–9. https://doi.org/10.1007/s00059-021-05076-5.
58. Dusi V, Angelini F, Zile MR, De Ferrari GM. Neuromodulation devices for heart failure Abstract Eur. Heart J Supp. 2022;24(Supplement_E):E12–E27. https://doi.org/10.1093/eurheartjsupp/suac036.
59. Giannino G, Nocera L, Andolfatto M, Braia V, Giacobbe F, Bruno F, et al. Vagal nerve stimulation in myocardial ischemia/reperfusion injury: from bench to bedside. Abstract BM. 2024;10(1). https://doi.org/10.1186/s42234-024-00153-6.
60. Schwartz PJ, De Ferrari GM. Sympathetic-parasympathetic interaction in health and disease: abnormalities and relevance in heart failure. Heart Fail Rev. 2011;16:101–7. https://doi.org/10.1007/s10741-010-9179-1.
61. Cardiac Sympathetic-Parasympathetic Interaction JACC: Basic to Translational Science. 2020;5(8):811–4. https://doi.org/10.1016/j.jacbts.2020.07.004.

62. Chin A, Ntsekhe M, Viljoen C, Rossouw J, Pennel T, Schwartz PJ. Rationale and design of a prospective study to assess the effect of left cardiac sympathetic denervation in chronic heart failure. Int J Cardiol. 2017;248:227–31. https://doi.org/10.1016/j.ijcard.2017.08.012.
63. Geis WP, Kaye MP, Randall WC. Major autonomic pathways to the atria and S-A and A-V nodes in the canine heart. Am J Phys. 1973;224:202–8. https://doi.org/10.1152/ajplegacy.1973.224.1.202.
64. Leftheriotis D, Flevari P, Kossyvakis C, Katsaras D, Batistaki C, Arvaniti C, et al. Acute effects of unilateral temporary stellate ganglion block on human atrial electrophysiological properties and atrial fibrillation inducibility. Heart Rhythm. 2016;13:2111–7. https://doi.org/10.1016/j.hrthm.2016.06.025.
65. Prognostic impact of atrial rhythm and dimension in patients with structural heart disease undergoing cardiac sympathetic denervation for ventricular arrhythmias. Heart Rhythm. 2020;17(5):714–20. https://doi.org/10.1016/j.hrthm.2019.12.007.
66. Randall WC, Armour JA, Geis WP, Lippincott DB. Regional cardiac distribution of the sympathetic nerves. Fed Proc. 1972;31:1199–208.
67. Kralios FA, Martin L, Burgess MJ, Millar K. Local ventricular repolarization changes due to sympathetic nerve-branch stimulation. Am J Phys. 1975;228:1621–6. https://doi.org/10.1152/ajplegacy.1975.228.5.1621.
68. Goodall M, Kirshner N. Effect of cervico-thoracic ganglionectomy on the adrenaline and noradrenaline content in the mammalian heart. J Clin Invest. 1956;35:649–56.
69. Hertting G, Schlefthaler TH. The effect of stellate ganglion excision on the catecholamine content and the uptake of 3H-norepinephrine in the heart of the cat. Int J Neuro-Oncol. 1964;3:65–9.
70. Schwartz PJ, Stone HL. Left stellectomy and denervation supersensitivity in conscious dogs. Am J Cardiol. 1982;49:1185–90. https://doi.org/10.1016/0002-9149(82)90043-1.
71. Dusi V, De Ferrari GM, Pugliese L, Schwartz PJ. Cardiac sympathetic denervation in channelopathies. Front Cardiovasc Med. 2019;6:27. https://doi.org/10.3389/fcvm.2019.00027.

Part II

Stellate Ganglion Block and Ventricular Arrhythmias

The Rationale for the Percutaneous Stellate Ganglion Block

4

Enrico Baldi, Sara Compagnoni,
Francesca Romana Gentile, and Simone Savastano

In the previous chapter, we illustrated the autonomic nervous system and its electrophysiological effects, emphasizing the significant role of the sympathetic system in the initiation and maintenance of ventricular arrhythmias.

In the present chapter, we will provide a practical overview of the stellate ganglion block and explore its role in the management of patients with therapy-resistant ventricular arrythmias.

We will examine two distinct patient groups: those who have experienced cardiac arrest and those with recurrent ventricular tachycardia or ventricular fibrillation (VF) and no cardiac arrest.

Patients with Cardiac Arrest: The Importance of Reducing the Number of Defibrillations

Treatment protocols of patients with cardiac arrest are guided by the European Resuscitation Council (ERC) [1] and the American Heart Association (AHA) [2] guidelines, which recommend rhythm assessment and defibrillation every 2 min for shockable rhythm, alongside drug therapy using amiodarone or lidocaine—these drugs share the indications and the class of recommendation. Refractory VF, although lacking of a universally accepted definition, is often described as VF persisting despite more than three shocks and the administration of 300 mg of amiodarone [3]; other authors suggest considering five shocks [4].

(translated by Chiara Barbaglia)

E. Baldi (✉) · S. Compagnoni · F. R. Gentile · S. Savastano
Division of Cardiology, Arrhythmology and Electrophysiology Unit,
Fondazione IRCCS Policlinico San Matteo, Pavia, Italy
e-mail: enrico.baldi@unipv.it

S. Savastano (ed.), *Percutaneous Stellate Ganglion Block for Electrical Storm*,
https://doi.org/10.1007/978-3-031-81762-5_4

The incidence of refractory VF varies widely in literature, ranging between 4% [5] and 10% [4], reflecting the absence of a standardized definition. Prognosis for refractory VF is generally poor, and the possible strategies [3] beside the Advanced Cardiac Life Support algorithm are limited. Studies demonstrated that survival rates at 1 month after cardiac arrest dramatically decline with increasing numbers of delivered shocks (Fig. 4.1).

An interesting study by Hasegawa et al. on OHCA patients 1 month after the event showed that those who received more than three pre-hospital defibrillations had a higher likelihood of death [6].

Subsequently, a study by Holmén et al. corroborated this finding, demonstrating that a higher number of defibrillations correlated with increased mortality at 1 month after OHCA, regardless of whether the cardiac arrest was witnessed or not: chances of survival significantly declined after the first three shocks with less pronounced reduction observed after ten or more shocks [7]. The relationship between survival and the number of defibrillations can be explained: during cardiac arrest, the blood flow is provided solely by cardiopulmonary resuscitation (CPR) which typically generates only the 25% of the normal cardiac output when performed correctly [8]. As the duration of cardiac arrest increases, so does the number of required shocks and the duration of the hypoperfusion phase, which negatively impact survival.

Furthermore, myocardial damage induced by defibrillation, the persistence of VF, and reperfusion injury all contribute significantly to the pathogenesis of cardiac dysfunction post-resuscitation from cardiac arrest [9, 10]. Medical literature has by now largely demonstrated the correlation between the total electrical energy

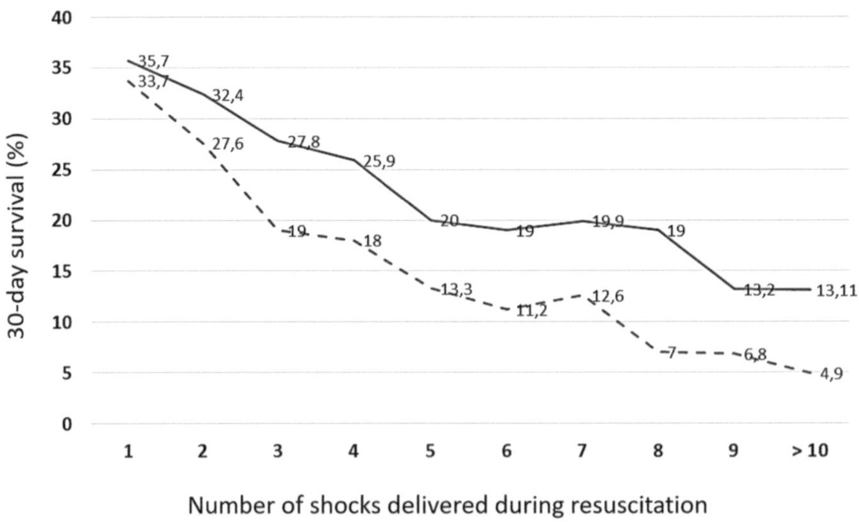

Fig. 4.1 Reduction of survival at 30 days after out-of-hospital cardiac arrest (OHCA) in function of the number of shocks delivered during resuscitation. Continuous blue line, data of the study by Hasegawa and colleagues [6]; dotted orange line, data of the study by Holmén et al. [7]

delivered during defibrillations and myocardial impairment [11, 12]. For instance, Xie J et al. showed how post-resuscitation myocardial disfunction and survival depend on the total amount of electrical energy delivered during defibrillation on mouse models [13]. The damage inflicted on the myocardium by repeated shocks [14], especially in case of refractory or recurrent VF, underscores the need for new strategies to minimize the number of defibrillations [15]. Besides, failure in early termination of ventricular fibrillations perpetuates a vicious cycle: as the heart exhausts its energy to maintain its electrical activity, the amplitude of ventricular fibrillation spectral area (AMSA) decreases, thereby increasing resistance to defibrillation attempts [16] and leading to asystolia [17].

Accumulation of intracellular calcium during prolonged VF, together with myocardial ischemia, results in mechanical changes. Studies using magnetic resonance (MR) on swine models induced into VF have identified three phases of cardiac arrest: an electrical phase, occurring within the first 5 min of the cardiac arrest, where arterial blood pressure remains higher than central venous pressure; a circulatory phase occurring from 5 to 15 min after the onset of the arrhythmia, when arterial blood and central venous pressures equalize, and a metabolic phase, starting 15 min after the cardiac arrest, marked by significant cellular alterations. The first mechanical changes occur within the first minutes of the electrical phase with rapid dilatation of the right ventricle; during the circulatory and metabolic phases, left ventricular wall thickness progressively increases due to myocardial edema, resulting in a loss of left ventricular intracavitary volume and gradually developing the so-called stone heart (Fig. 4.2).

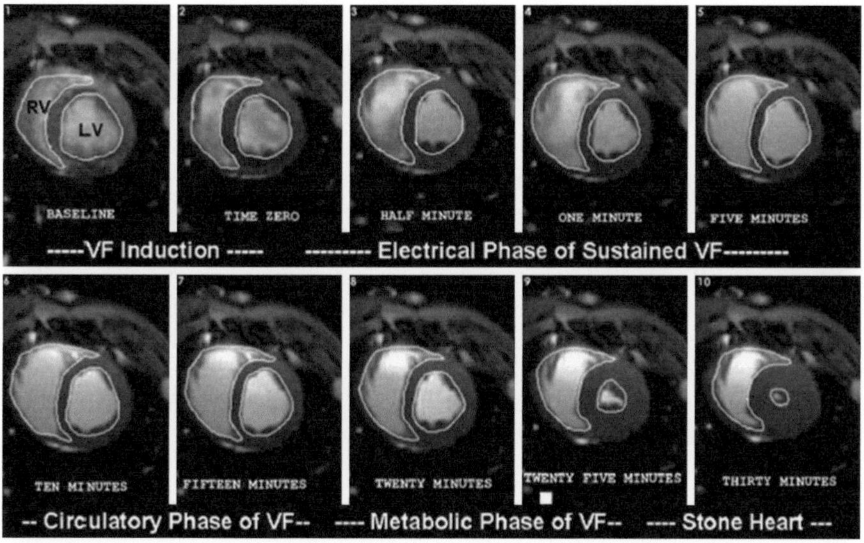

Fig. 4.2 Images of short axes of the right and left ventricles during 30 min of sustained VF in a swine model. The endocardial edge is delineated. Baseline, sinus rhythm. Time zero, onset of ventricular fibrillation (from Sorrell VL et al. Resuscitation. 2007;73:279–286) [18]

In the initial minutes following the onset of VF—electrical phase—hemodynamic conditions remain favorable and similar to the physiologic state: defibrillation during this period will result in better chances of restoring spontaneous circulation compared to attempts made after 25–30 min of cardiac arrest. Furthermore, the hypoperfusion time between the onset of VF and the restoration of spontaneous circulation may predispose to reperfusion injury, the severity of which depends on the total duration of the ischemia [19].

Therefore, prompt restoration of spontaneous heart rhythm must be the primary goal in managing cardiac arrest.

Patients with Arrhythmias without Cardiac Arrest: Terminating the Electrical Storm Using the Minimum of Electrical Shocks

The restoration of spontaneous rhythm remains the priority for patients with electrical storm, even if they have not cardiac arrest, in order to improve outcomes.

Many of these patients already have implantable cardioverter defibrillators (ICDs). Despite the very short hypoperfusion time due to the rapid and effective ICD therapy within few seconds from the onset of the arrhythmia, survival rates decline as the number of received shocks increases, whether delivered by a manual external defibrillator or from an ICD [20, 21]. Repeated defibrillations from either device type are associated with reduced long-term survival compared to patients who have never received any shock.

Studies by Pacifico and by McIntyre [20, 21] demonstrated that multiple electrical shocks represent a mortality risk factor and introduced the idea of cardiac impairment caused by cumulative shocks.

Conversely, the use of anti-tachycardia pacing (ATP) alone for treating ventricular arrhythmias has not shown an association with increased mortality. In ATP therapy, the ICD delivers electrical stimulation at a higher frequency than the ongoing tachycardia without administering any electrical shock, thereby preserving cardiac function from impairment and reducing the risk of negative outcomes [21–23]. Unfortunately, as described by Hayashi et al. [23], only half patients with electrical storm (ES) benefit from ATP therapy and in patients with a history of ES [24], ICD programming typically involves a more aggressive therapy with fewer ATPs and earlier shocks. Therefore, proper device programming [25] and effective reduction of arrhythmias are crucial in minimizing the number of electrical shocks.

The autonomic nervous system plays a central role both in initiating and maintaining the electrical storm: Fig. 4.3 depicts the "vicious cycle" of ventricular arrhythmias deteriorating into electrical storm [26].

Rapid ventricular tachycardia or ventricular fibrillation causes a sudden decrease in cardiac output and, consequently, blood pressure. To restore adequate cardiac

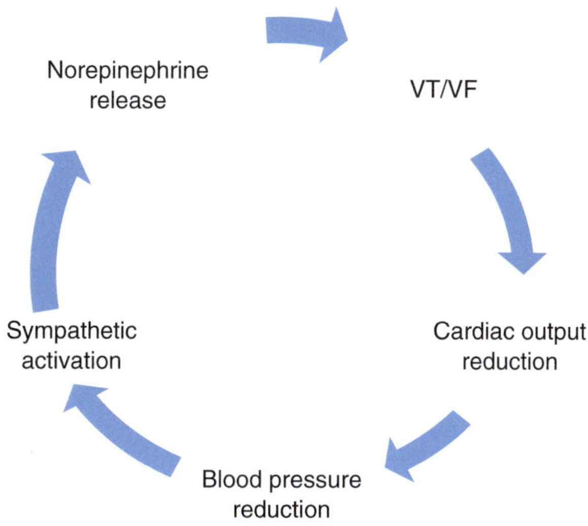

Fig. 4.3 The vicious cycle of the electrical storm

function, the sympathetic nervous system releases noradrenaline into the myocardium; noradrenaline, in turn (Chap. 3), triggers ventricular arrhythmias perpetuating the vicious arrhythmic cycle (Fig. 4.3).

The effectiveness of the percutaneous stellate ganglion block (PSGB) in interrupting electrical storm underscores the central role of the autonomic nervous system. Although PSGB has a temporary duration by definition, in most patients, arrhythmias do not recur after the procedure ends, halting the vicious cycle. Comorbidities that persist after the end of the anesthetic effect, such as sepsis or hyperthyroidism, can hinder immediate arrhythmia resolution. Nevertheless, many studies including our own experience demonstrate that a single PSGB with bolus administration has been sufficient to stop electrical storm, minimizing the need for repeated procedures or continuous infusion.

Traditional therapies for electrical storm are not always promptly effective and may induce hypotension (i.e., intravenous amiodarone [27–29]) or depress myocardial contractility (i.e., certain antiarrhythmic drugs [30] or high-dosage beta-blockers), triggering the sympathetic system.

Amiodarone and lidocaine, followed by procainamide and sotalol, are the most used, particularly in the treatment of structural heart disease. A small American case study reports amiodarone as the most effective therapy for shock-resistant VF, albeit with a 50% efficacy rate [31]. Besides, Levine et al. note a slow onset of action of amiodarone, with a 20% efficacy rate after 2 h from administration [32].

Therefore, percutaneous ganglion block therapy may play a more decisive role in managing patients with electrical storm.

References

1. Soar J, Böttiger BW, Carli P, et al. European resuscitation council guidelines 2021: adult advanced life support. Resuscitation. 2021;161:115–51. https://doi.org/10.1016/j.resuscitation.2021.02.010.
2. Panchal AR, Bartos JA, Cabañas JG, et al. Part 3: adult basic and advanced life support: 2020 American Heart Association Guidelines for Cardiopulmonary Resuscitation and Emergency Cardiovascular Care. Circulation. 2020;142(16_2):S366–468. https://doi.org/10.1161/CIR.0000000000000916.
3. Yannopoulos D, Bartos JA, Martin C, et al. Minnesota resuscitation consortium's advanced perfusion and reperfusion cardiac life support strategy for out-of-hospital refractory ventricular fibrillation. J Am Heart Assoc. 2016;5:6. https://doi.org/10.1161/JAHA.116.003732.
4. Hira RS, Nichol G. Management of refractory ventricular fibrillation: extracorporeal membrane oxygenation or epinephrine? JACC Basic Transl Sci. 2017;2(3):254–7. https://doi.org/10.1016/J.JACBTS.2017.04.001.
5. Bell SM, Lam DH, Kearney K, Hira RS. Management of refractory ventricular fibrillation (prehospital and emergency department). Cardiol Clin. 2018;36(3):395–408. https://doi.org/10.1016/J.CCL.2018.03.007.
6. Hasegawa M, Abe T, Nagata T, Onozuka D, Hagihara A. The number of prehospital defibrillation shocks and 1-month survival in patients with out-of-hospital cardiac arrest. Scand J Trauma Resusc Emerg Med. 2015;23:1. https://doi.org/10.1186/s13049-015-0112-4.
7. Holmén J, Hollenberg J, Claesson A, et al. Survival in ventricular fibrillation with emphasis on the number of defibrillations in relation to other factors at resuscitation. Resuscitation. 2017;113:33–8. https://doi.org/10.1016/J.RESUSCITATION.2017.01.006.
8. Sandroni C, De Santis P, D'Arrigo S. Capnography during cardiac arrest. Resuscitation. 2018;132:73–7. https://doi.org/10.1016/J.RESUSCITATION.2018.08.018.
9. Gazmuri RJ, Weil MH, Bisera J, Tang W, Fukui M, McKee D. Myocardial dysfunction after successful resuscitation from cardiac arrest. Crit Care Med. 1996;24(6):992–1000. https://doi.org/10.1097/00003246-199606000-00020.
10. Kern KB, Hilwig RW, Rhee KH, Berg RA. Myocardial dysfunction after resuscitation from cardiac arrest: an example of global myocardial stunning. J Am Coll Cardiol. 1996;28(1):232–40. https://doi.org/10.1016/0735-1097(96)00130-1.
11. Tang W, Weil MH, Sun S. Low-energy biphasic waveform defibrillation reduces the severity of postresuscitation myocardial dysfunction. Crit Care Med. 2000;28(11 Suppl) https://doi.org/10.1097/00003246-200011001-00014.
12. Huang J, Ruse RB, Walcott GP, et al. Ascending defibrillation waveform significantly reduces myocardial morphological damage and injury current. JACC Clin Electrophysiol. 2019;5(7):854–62. https://doi.org/10.1016/J.JACEP.2019.04.006.
13. Xie J, Weil MH, Sun S, et al. High-energy defibrillation increases the severity of postresuscitation myocardial dysfunction. Circulation. 1997;96(2):683–8. https://doi.org/10.1161/01.CIR.96.2.683.
14. Walcott GP, Killingsworth CR, Ideker RE. Do clinically relevant transthoracic defibrillation energies cause myocardial damage and dysfunction? Resuscitation. 2003;59(1):59–70. https://doi.org/10.1016/S0300-9572(03)00161-8.
15. Gazmuri RJ. Effects of repetitive electrical shocks on postresuscitation myocardial function. Crit Care Med. 2000;28(11 Suppl) https://doi.org/10.1097/00003246-200011001-00016.
16. Frigerio L, Baldi E, Aramendi E, et al. End-tidal carbon dioxide (ETCO2) and ventricular fibrillation amplitude spectral area (AMSA) for shock outcome prediction in out-of-hospital cardiac arrest. Are they two sides of the same coin? Resuscitation. 2021;160:142–9. https://doi.org/10.1016/J.RESUSCITATION.2020.10.032.
17. Kern KB, Garewal HS, Sanders AB, et al. Depletion of myocardial adenosine triphosphate during prolonged untreated ventricular fibrillation: effect on defibrillation success. Resuscitation. 1990;20(3):221–9. https://doi.org/10.1016/0300-9572(90)90005-Y.

18. Sorrell VL, Bhatt RD, Berg RA, et al. Cardiac magnetic resonance imaging investigation of sustained ventricular fibrillation in a swine model—with a focus on the electrical phase. Resuscitation. 2007;73(2):279–86. https://doi.org/10.1016/J.RESUSCITATION.2006.08.032.
19. Leistner M, Sommer S, Kanofsky P, Leyh R, Sommer SP. Ischemia time impacts on respiratory chain functions and Ca 2+-handling of cardiac subsarcolemmal mitochondria subjected to ischemia reperfusion injury. J Cardiothorac Surg. 2019;14:1. https://doi.org/10.1186/S13019-019-0911-1.
20. Pacifico A, Ferlic LL, Cedillo-Salazar FER, Nasir N, Doyle TK, Henry PD. Shocks as predictors of survival in patients with implantable cardioverter-defibrillators. J Am Coll Cardiol. 1999;34(1):204–10. https://doi.org/10.1016/S0735-1097(99)00142-4.
21. MacIntyre CJ, Sapp JL, Abdelwahab A, et al. The effect of shock burden on heart failure and mortality. CJC Open. 2019;1(4):161–7. https://doi.org/10.1016/J.CJCO.2019.04.003.
22. Strickberger SA, Canby R, Cooper J, et al. Association of antitachycardia pacing or shocks with survival in 69,000 patients with an implantable defibrillator. J Cardiovasc Electrophysiol. 2017;28(4):416–22. https://doi.org/10.1111/jce.13170.
23. Hayashi H, Shimizu W, Iwasaki Y, et al. Efficacy of antitachycardia pacing for electrical storms in patients with implantable defibrillators. J Cardiovasc Electrophysiol. 2021;32(3):823–31. https://doi.org/10.1111/JCE.14891.
24. Guerra F, Palmisano P, Dell'Era G, et al. Implantable cardioverter-defibrillator programming and electrical storm: results of the OBSERVational registry on long-term outcome of ICD patients (OBSERVO-ICD). Heart Rhythm. 2016;13(10):1987–92. https://doi.org/10.1016/J.HRTHM.2016.06.007.
25. Bennett MT, Brown ML, Koehler J, Lexcen DR, Cheng A, Cheung JW. Trends in implantable cardioverter-defibrillator programming practices and its impact on therapies: insights from a North American Remote Monitoring Registry 2007–2018. Heart Rhythm. Published online. 2021; https://doi.org/10.1016/J.HRTHM.2021.10.010.
26. Elsokkari I, Tsuji Y, Sapp JL, Nattel S. Recent insights into mechanisms and clinical approaches to electrical storm. Can J Cardiol . Published online January. 2022;1 https://doi.org/10.1016/J.CJCA.2021.12.015.
27. Kowey PR, Marinchak RA, Rials SJ, Filart RA. Intravenous amiodarone. J Am Coll Cardiol. 1997;29(6):1190–8. https://doi.org/10.1016/S0735-1097(97)00069-7.
28. Cushing DJ, Cooper WD, Gralinski MR, Lipicky RJ. The hypotensive effect of intravenous amiodarone is sustained throughout the maintenance infusion period. Clin Exp Pharmacol Physiol. 2010;37(3):358–61. https://doi.org/10.1111/J.1440-1681.2009.05303.X.
29. Doshi D, Jayawardana R. Amiodarone-induced life-threatening refractory hypotension. Am J Case Rep. 2015;16:617–20. https://doi.org/10.12659/AJCR.893920.
30. Schlepper M. Cardiodepressive effects of antiarrhythmic drugs. Eur Heart J. 1989;10(SUPPL. E):73–80. https://doi.org/10.1093/EURHEARTJ/10.SUPPL_E.73.
31. Somberg JC, Bailin SJ, Haffajee CI, et al. Intravenous lidocaine versus intravenous amiodarone (in a new aqueous formulation) for incessant ventricular tachycardia. Am J Cardiol. 2002;90(8):853–9. https://doi.org/10.1016/S0002-9149(02)02707-8.
32. Levine JH, Massumi A, Scheinman MM, et al. Intravenous amiodarone for recurrent sustained hypotensive ventricular tachyarrhythmias. J Am Coll Cardiol. 1996;27(1):67–75. https://doi.org/10.1016/0735-1097(95)00427-0.

Efficacy and Safety Data

5

S. Savastano, Francesca Romana Gentile, and Sara Compagnoni

For more than one century, sympathetic ganglion block has been an essential component in the multimodal treatment of neuropathic pain syndromes. Albeit it diverges from the primary focus of the present textbook, we should not overlook the percutaneous stellate ganglion block (PSGB) used for antalgic purpose considering that evidences and cases of its application over the years have provided data about safety, technical skills and equipment necessary for its application. The adaptation of PSGB for treating ventricular arrhythmias prompted the search for new and different evidence on effectiveness and methods of the procedure in this new context of arrhythmic storm.

The treatment of electrical storm (AS) ranges from pharmacological therapy (antiarrhythmic drugs and beta-blockers) to device reprogramming or cardiac sympathetic denervation (CSD) and catheter ablation. These therapies might not always be readily available in all hospitals or sufficient to solve the high-mortality condition of AS. Timely intervention is crucial in resolving of AS or cardiac arrest. Once all the main potential causes (metabolic disorders, electrolyte abnormalities, drug adverse effects or myocardial ischaemia) have been identified and all the available therapies administered, a rapid and straightforward procedure is needed to stabilise the patients before transferring them to a specialised centre for a definitive treatment.

Studies by Schwartz [1] and Malliani [2] on the role of sympathetic autonomic nervous system in the triggering and maintenance of ventricular arrhythmias

---

The original version of the chapter has been revised. A correction to this chapter can be found at https://doi.org/10.1007/978-3-031-81762-5_11

(translated by Chiara Barbaglia)

S. Savastano (✉) · F. R. Gentile · S. Compagnoni
Division of Cardiology, Arrhythmology and Electrophysiology Unit, Fondazione IRCCS Policlinico San Matteo, Pavia, Italy
e-mail: S.Savastano@smatteo.pv.it

S. Savastano (ed.), *Percutaneous Stellate Ganglion Block for Electrical Storm*, https://doi.org/10.1007/978-3-031-81762-5_5

highlighted cardiac sympathetic neuromodulation as a valid therapeutic option to reduce myocardial susceptibility to ventricular fibrillation. Beside beta-blocker therapy, thoracic epidural anaesthesia (TEA) and PSGB are recognised as the most effective methods to determine temporary cardiac neuromodulation. While TEA presents a series of limitations, including the risk of epidural hematoma in patients on anticoagulation therapy, requirement for specialised medical equipment, higher expertise in technical skills and patient positioning (sitting or lying on the side), PSGB is a less invasive procedure. It can be performed at the patient's bedside, requiring little and low-cost equipment without the need for sedation or interruption of anticoagulation therapy and without interfering with resuscitation manoeuvres.

Reports evaluating the effectiveness of PSGB are not few but exhibit considerable variability. Moreover, most studies are monocentric, retrospective and non-randomised and involve small samples size, predominantly on adult population. Despite the heterogeneity in clinical contexts, techniques and outcome metrics, a common thread of evidence support the inclusion of PSGB in the list of clinical practices for the management of refractory electrical storm.

Case Reports on Adult Patients

The first clinical report—published by Grossman [3] in New York in 1976—describes the case of a 56-year-old woman with intracerebral haemorrhage from ruptured basilar artery aneurysm. During hospitalisation, the patient had drug-resistant VT (lidocaine, phenytoin, atropine, procainamide digoxin and propranolol), and the admission ECG showed a prolonged QT of 640 msec.

Based on the studies on ECG abnormalities in patients with central nervous system disease [4] and on the role of left cardiac sympathetic denervation (LCSD) in shortening the QT interval in a patient with idiopathic and drug-resistant LQTS [5], PSGB was performed with the injection of 15 ml 1% lidocaine into the region of the left stellate ganglion block. The procedure stopped both ventricular arrhythmias and repolarisation abnormalities, after which the patient underwent neurosurgical intervention.

The first Italian case report dates back to the 1980s: Biagini et al. [6], following the experimental studies by Schwartz [1], performed PSGB on a 58-year-old patient on the eighth day after acute myocardial infarction in order to stop the multiple episodes of VF. By injecting 120 mg lidocaine into the left stellate ganglion, Biagini managed to stop ventricular arrhythmias which did not respond to intravenous lidocaine and recurred with each electric shock. Together with the restoration of normal heart rhythm, left palpebral ptosis occurred. Supposing that a longer half-life drug could prolong the antiarrhythmic effect, a subsequent PSGB using mepivacaine was performed after a second block with lidocaine. Mepivacaine PSGB was repeated twice within 36 h; ocular signs were monitored; rare ventricular ectopic beats and no arrhythmia were observed. Although neither Grossman nor Biagini gave precise details regarding the technique used, it is reasonably to presume they applied the anatomic technique (Table 5.1).

In 2013, Hayase et al. described the case of an 80-year-old man with ICD and post-ischaemic dilated hypokinetic heart disease with prior surgical myocardial

Table 5.1 The main characteristics of the clinical cases where PSGB was performed

Author	Year	Background of the electrical storm	Anaesthetic used	Technique	Side	Effectiveness	Complications
Grossman et al. [3]	1976	Rupture of cerebral aneurysm in a healthy heart	Lidocaine	Not described	Left	Yes	No
Biagini et al. [6]	1985	Subacute myocardial infarction	Lidocaine and mepivacaine	Not described	Left	Yes	No
Hoepp ed. t al [7].	1990	Long QT syndrome	Mepivacaine	Not described	Left	Yes	No
Patel et al. [8]	2011	72 h post-BPAC	Unknown	At the level of C7 but not described the technique	Left	Yes	No
Loyalka et al. [9]	2011	STEMI	Bupivacaine	Frontal-anatomical	Left	Yes	No
Tan et al. [10]	2012	Post-myocardial dilated hypokinetic heart disease, FE 15%.	Bupivacaine	Antero-lateral paratracheal approach Under fluoroscopic guidance	Left	Yes	No
Hayase et al. [11]	2013	Post-ischaemic dilated hypokinetic heart disease, FE 30%	Bupivacaine	At T1 level under fluoroscopic guidance	Alternating left and right	Yes	No
Garcia et al. [12]	2013	STEMI complicated by decompensation	Bupivacaine	Front	Left	Yes	No
Gadhinglajkar et al. [13]	2013	Post-infarct CMD	Bupivacaine	Only described as echo-driven	Left	Yes	No
Mata et al. [14]	2014	STEMI and cardiogenic shock	Bupivacaine and ropivacaine	Front	Left	Yes	No
Malik et al. [15]	2014	Post-ischaemic CMD	Bupivacaine	Lateral under fluoroscopic guidance at the level of C6	Left	Yes	No

(continued)

Table 5.1 (continued)

Author	Year	Background of the electrical storm	Anaesthetic used	Technique	Side	Effectiveness	Complications
Hulata et al. [16]	2015	Post-ischaemic CMD on BPAC outcomes	Ropivacaine	Ultrasound-guided lateral	Left	Yes	No
Scanlon et al. [17]	2015	96 hours post-BPAC. In ECO for refractory cardiac arrest	Bupivacaine	Lateral ultrasound	Left and right simultaneously	Yes	No
Smith et al. [18]	2015	Non-ischaemic CMD carrying VAD	Lidocaine	Lateral ultrasound-guided (inter-vascular)	Left	Yes	No
Fudim et al. [19]	2017	Non-ischaemic CMD	Lidocaine	Anterior Ultrasound-guided at C7 level	Left and right	Yes	No
		Post-BPAC	Bupivacaine	Anterior ultrasound at C7 level	Left and right	Yes	No
Przybylski at al [20]	2018	Post-ischaemic CMD	Lidocaine	Only described as ultrasound-guided	Left	Yes	No
		Post-ischaemic CMD	Lidocaine	Only described as ultrasound-guided	Right and left	Yes	No
Yang et al. [21]	2019	Non-ischaemic CMD; amiodarone thyrotoxicosis	Lidocaine and bupivacaine	Lateral ultrasound-guided	Left	Yes	No

Savastano et al. [22]	2020	Post-ischaemic CMD	Lidocaine and bupivacaine	Anatomical frontal	Left	Yes	No
Savastano et al. [23]	2020	Anterior STEMI. On ECMO for refractory arrest	Lidocaine and Bupivacaine	Anatomical frontal	Left	Yes	No
Sahoo et al. [24]	2021	Post-infarct CMD	Bupivacaine	Lateral ultrasound-guided with patient in right lateral decubitus	Left	Yes	No
		Post-infarct CMD	Bupivacaine	Lateral ultrasound-guided with patient in right lateral decubitus	Left	Yes	No
		Non-ischaemic CMD	Bupivacaine	Lateral ultrasound-guided with patient in right lateral decubitus	Left	Yes	No
Pillai et al. [25]	2021	Long QT	Bupivacaine	Frontal ultrasound-guided	Left and right	Yes	Laryngeal nerve palsy
Mohd et al. [26]	2021	Acute AMI	Lidocaine	Lateral ultrasound-guided at C7 level	Left	Yes	No

List of clinical cases on stellate ganglion block in adult patients with electrical storm
CABG coronary artery bypass graft, *STEMI* ST elevation myocardial infarction, *DCM* dilated cardiomyopathy, *HCM* hypertrophic cardiomyopathy, *ECMO* extracorporeal membrane oxygenation, *VAD* ventricular assist device

revascularisation, who presented at the emergency department after multiple ICD shocks. The patient had sotalol, mexiletine and carvedilol administered and was intolerant to amiodarone. He had previously undergone two endocardial and one epicardial ablations but had been ineligible for left cardiac sympathetic denervation (LCSD) owing to pleuro-pericardial adhesions resulting from prior coronary artery bypass surgery. The patient underwent PSGB twice a week, alternating between left ganglion and right ganglion blocks to minimise respiratory complications associated with potential bilateral damage of the recurrent laryngeal nerve or of the phrenic nerve. This treatment continued for 4 weeks. No further ICD shock was registered at the follow-up.

Based on the efficacy of bilateral denervation [27], in 2015, Scanlon et al. [17] described the case of a 79-year-old woman with refractory AS receiving extracorporeal membrane oxygenation (ECMO) and intra-aortic balloon pump (IABP) therapy who underwent bilateral percutaneous stellate ganglion block (PSGB). PSGB was chosen in the hypothesis of a greater antiarrhythmic efficacy for the patient as she was already in tracheal intubation (i.e. at lower risk of complications from bilateral paralysis of the laryngeal or phrenic nerve) and had a severe haemodynamic instability.

In the same year, Smith et al. [18] treated a 65-years-old with left assisting ventricular device (LVAD) and ICD in electrical storm (12 VT with 12 shocks in 24 h) using inter-vascular ultrasound-guided PSGB, administered as both bolus and several-day-lasting infusion. Both medical therapy (mexiletine, amiodarone and metoprolol) and trans-catheter ablation had failed; heart transplantation had been excluded owing to oncological disease. Given the multiple shocks delivered by the ICD (>3 per day), LSCD considered the only viable option, although with a high anaesthesiologic risk. In this case, PSGB was applied as a *trial* before surgical denervation. The case study stands out both for the innovative technique—inserting the needle between the left carotid artery and the left jugular vein—and for the use of PSGB as trial for assessing the potential success of cardiac denervation. After the antiarrhythmic effect of the PSGB, the patient successfully underwent LSCD on the seventh day.

Pillai et al. [25] describe the case of a 60-year-old patient with cardiac arrest with return of spontaneous circulation, presenting with prolonged QT interval. He had in-hospital AS on day three despite medical treatment with beta-blockers, lidocaine and deep sedation. PSGB successfully treated recurrent ventricular arrhythmias, although vocal paralysis and respiratory distress occurred shortly after the procedure, necessitating intubation. Left recurrent laryngeal nerve paralysis resolved spontaneously in hospital on day 6th. The patient underwent bilateral surgical sympathetic denervation and ICD implantation and was discharged on nadolol. The 6-month-follow -up did not reveal any recurrence of arrhythmias. In spite of the occurrence of a temporary complication from the procedure, this case underscores the effectiveness of PSGB treatment in AS and its role in evaluating the potential success of surgical denervation.

In a 2021 study by Mohd and colleagues [26], a 42-year-old man with acute myocardial infarction experienced three episodes of in-hospital cardiac arrest.

PSGB was performed following systemic thrombolysis; no complications occurred, and ventricular arrhythmias were suppressed for 30 h.

The following cases belong to our experience and differ from the ones described above for the exclusive execution of left PSGB using the anterior anatomy-guided approach according to the modified Moore's technique. One case involved a 62-year-old patient with electrical storm refractory to direct current shock, antiarrhythmic therapy combined with esmolol infusion, sedation and intubation. We performed a series of single blocks with anterior anatomically guided approach followed by continuous infusion (2% lidocaine) via a common epidural catheter. Based on the positive response to PSGB, subsequent cardiac sympathectomy was then successfully performed resulting in complete suppression of ventricular arrhythmias during follow-up.

Another case involved a woman with cardiac arrest due to persistent ventricular fibrillation during ECMO placement. After one PSGB with lidocaine, heart rhythm was restored and coronary reperfusion performed in the cath lab. Following a primary coronary intervention on the proximal left anterior descendant artery, a second PSGB was performed (lidocaine and bupivacaine) due to the recurrence of VF, suppressing the arrhythmia. Despite the challenges posed by the anticoagulation and double antiplatelet therapies (due to the ECMO and the percutaneous revascularisation), the anatomically guided approach of PSGB procedure was proved to be both safe and effective.

Observations: despite the diversity of the clinical settings, PSGB consistently led to a rapid haemodynamic stabilisation of the patients, guiding them toward a more definitive therapy (ICD implantation, LCSD, trans-catheter ablation, heart transplantation). In some rare cases, where other options were contraindicated, PSGB worked as a viable alternative therapy. Interestingly, the duration of PSGB effect varied broadly, regardless of the anaesthetic drugs used, confirming the coexistence of two distinct effects of PSGB: an acute anaesthetic effect and a long-lasting one, consisting in the remodelling of neural structures, nerve fibres and ganglia and cardiac substrate.

Both the approach (single, daily, biweekly block, continuous infusion) and technique (anatomic, ultrasound-guided, fluoroscopic) of the PSGB vary widely.

Clearly, due to the nature of individual case studies, the cases described above neither provide definitive conclusions on the effectiveness of the left stellate ganglion block nor confirm the hypothetical additional benefits of the right or bilateral stellate ganglion block.

Markers of complete PSGB—vasodilatation leading to temperature rise, asthenia of the ipsilateral upper limb and Horner syndrome characterised by palpebral ptosis, myosis and anhidrosis—were detailed in only few of the above studies. These manifestations may not be specific or sensitive for several reasons: (1) the sympathetic eye fibres run in the superior section of the stellate ganglion and in the medium and superior cervical ganglia, (2) some patients can be intubated or sedated, and (3) the low flow during cardiac arrest or ventricular arrhythmias leads to vasoconstriction.

Case Reports on Paediatric Patients

Paediatric case reports of PSGB mostly concern LQTS patients. In the late 1950s, the Jervell and Lange-Nielsen syndrome [28] and subsequently the Romano-Ward syndrome (RWS) [29, 30] were first described, highlighting their association in sudden cardiac death. Following the first evidence of the effect of the stimulation of the sympathetic stellate ganglion on the QT interval, in the 1960s, a 12-year-old girl with RWS underwent PSGB resulting in successful QT interval shortening on baseline ECG and suppression of ventricular arrhythmias [31].

In 1991, Parris et al. [32] reported cases of PSGB using the anterior anatomically guided technique with bupivacaine in two children with different clinical conditions. In one of them, a 6-year-old girl with LQTS, the procedure was performed with antiarrhythmic purpose. Ventricular arrhythmias had resisted to both medical management with isoproterenol, bretylium and phenytoin and to 120 bpm pacing. To direct the patient to LCSD, PSGB with 5 ml bupivacaine (0.25%) was performed; this allowed to obtain haemodynamical stabilisation for 24 h and to stop VT adrenergic trigger, successfully performing LCDS.

In 1993, Mesa et al. [33] performed PSGB with 5 ml bupivacaine at 0.25% (0.34 mg/kg) to treat AS in a 9-year-old child with LQTS and insulin-dependent diabetes mellitus. Differently from the case described above, the catheter for the local anaesthetic was secured to the child's skin in order to repeat PSGB once the sympatholytic effects (different temperature between the left and right arm and variation in the pupil size) dissipated.

Finally, in 2019, Franklin et al. [34] described the case of a 6-year-old child with LQTS with recurrent episodes of polymorphic VT and ventricular fibrillation necessitating extracorporeal membrane oxygenation (ECMO) support. Despite the use of anticoagulation, ultrasound-guided PSGB procedure was performed with 0.5% lidocaine at 2 ml/h, successfully stopping VT and restoring sinus rhythm.

The only case of a paediatric patient with structural heart disease was described by Boe et al. [35] in 2012. In this case, PSGB not only stopped ventricular arrhythmias and reduced the number of ICD shocks in a 7-month-old infant, but it also facilitated LCSD before planning heart transplantation. Despite previous therapies with propranolol, amiodarone, esmolol, phosphophenytoin and verapamil failing to cease recurrent arrhythmias (resulting in two to three ICD shocks per day), lateral ultrasound-guided PSGB with 2 ml of 0.2% ropivacaine was successful. The baby underwent PSGB every day for a week; esmolol and lidocaine infusions were continued until LCSD, after which they were replaced by mexiletine and propranolol until heart transplantation. Histiocytoid cardiomyopathy was the final diagnosis.

Albeit the higher risk of complications due to ECMO or repeated PSGB procedures, these paediatric case reports demonstrate a high level of safety and effectiveness (Table 5.2) comparable to adult case reports.

Table 5.2 List of clinical cases on stellate ganglion block in paediatric patients with electrical storm

Author	Year	Background of the electrical storm	Anaesthetic used	Technique	Side	Effectiveness	Complications
Yanagida et al. [31]	1976	12-year-old girl with Romano-Ward syndrome	Lidocaine	Not described	Left	Yes, in QT interval shortening and arrhythmia suppressing	No
Parris et al. [32]	1991	6-year-old girl with long QT syndrome	Bupivacaine	Anterior anatomical	Left	Yes	No
Mesa et al. [33]	1993	9-year-old boy with long QT syndrome	Bupivacaine	Anterior anatomical	Left	Yes	No
Boe et al. [35]	2012	7-month-old baby with HCM	Ropivacaine	Lateral ultrasound-guided	Left	Yes	No
Frankling et al. [34]	2019	6-year-old girl with long QT syndrome on ECMO for refractory cardiac arrest	Lidocaine (infusion)	Anterior ultrasound-guided at C6 level	Left	Yes	No

HCM hypertrophic cardiomyopathy, *ECMO* extracorporeal membrane oxygenation

Observational Studies

In the recent years, some monocentric and retrospective studies involving consecutive patients and sometimes including control groups have been conducted in order to provide stronger evidence to the safety and effectiveness of PSGB.

In 2000, Nademanee et al. [36] first demonstrated that patients with myocardial infarction and AS treated with SNS block (esmolol, propranolol or PSGB) had a better outcome compared to those treated with antiarrhythmic drugs following ACLS guidelines. Forty-nine patients were divided into two groups: group 1 received SNS block treatment, and group 2 (control group) received standard ACLS treatment. Both short- and long-term mortality rates were higher in group 2. The study suggested that sympathetic block should be the preferred treatment for AS. However, potential biases include physician discretion in selecting treatment for both groups and the study's focus on acute post-myocardial infarction AS patients, with a median time of 12 days between arrhythmias and acute myocardial infarction.

The effectiveness of PSGB in combination with nifekalant (NIF), an IKr channel blocker and class III antiarrhythmic, was described in a Japanese study by Amino and colleagues in 2007 [37] in patients with refractory cardiac arrest. They enrolled 55 patients with out-of-hospital cardiac arrest (OHCA), 15 of whom were refractory to nifekalant, CPR and external defibrillation. Of these 15, 11 patients were treated with PSGB in combination with NIF and 64% of them achieved restoration of spontaneous sinus rhythm; 55% patients treated with PSGB and NIF survived, while all patients in the non-PSGB group died. This study, conducted in hospital on OHCA patients, could only evaluate the effectiveness of PSGB in association with NIF, a drug approved solely in Japan.

In a case study by Prabu et al. [38], 9 patients with structural heart disease and AS underwent surgical denervation with five of them successfully treated with ultrasound-guided PSGB. In 2016, Garcia et al. [39] assessed the effectiveness of PSGB in addition to conventional therapy in eight patients with structural heart disease (ischaemic, valvular, dilated) and polymorphic VT. All patients received ultrasound-guided PSGB and continuous infusion of 0.2% ropivacaine at 6–12 ml/h infusion rate. In the 24 h following PSGB, VT episodes significantly decreased in six out of eight patients: the two nonresponsive to PSGB underwent epidural thoracic anaesthesia. Despite a high mortality rate, only one patient died from arrhythmia.

A monocentric retrospective study by Tian et al. [40] in 2019 enrolled 30 patients with refractory AS. Both ultrasound-guided lateral (postero-anteriorly directed needle) and antero-lateral fluoroscopic approach were performed. Conscious or emergency patients (15/30) received left unilateral PSGB, while intubated patients or patients nonresponsive to PSGB within 10 minutes underwent bilateral PSGB with potential for repeated procedures upon relapse. The increase in temperature in the ipsilateral arm confirmed sympatholysis. Out of a total amount of 38 blocks, 28 were performed with bupivacaine, 4 with lidocaine alone and 6 with both (for a total volume of 6–12 ml). The effectiveness of the procedure was evaluated both in the short-term (24 and 72 h post-PSGB) and in the long term (5–57 months follow-up). Ventricular arrhythmias were completely suppressed 24 h after PSGB in 60% patients; a higher in-hospital mortality rate was observed in patients with relapses of arrhythmias within 24 h from the block (94.5% vs 50%, $p = 0.009$). After 72 h from the block, complete suppression of arrhythmias was achieved in 15/30 patients, with partial persistency in 6/30 patients. Among ICD carriers, the number of arrhythmic episodes, as well as of the shocks, significantly decreased (92% compared to baseline). No complications occurred. The above case study reports a small subset (15) of patients treated with left PSGB alone describing both ultrasound-guided and fluoroscopic approach without identifying a superior method of the two.

Fudim et al. [41] performed bilateral PSGB in 20 consecutive patients assessing the effectiveness of the procedure by comparing arrhythmic episodes and shocks over the 24 and 48 hours before and after the procedure. Both arrhythmic episodes and shocks significantly reduced over the 24 h (0 vs 4.5, $p < 0.001$, and 0 vs 2, $p = 0.002$) and the 48 h (0 vs 5.5, $p < 0.001$, and 0 vs 2.5, $p = 0.002$). A total of 45% patients experienced a complete response without recurrence of ventricular arrhythmias over 48 h after PSGB; 20% patients had no recurrence of VT upon discharge. Response rates were similar in patients with ischaemic (median 6 [IQR: 1.8–18.8] to 0.5 [IQR: 0–5.3] events; $p = 0.031$) and non-ischaemic cardiomyopathy (median 3.5 [IQR: 1.8–6.8] to 0 [IQR: 0–1.3] events; $p = 0.012$) and with monomorphic and polymorphic VT. A total of 60% patients were intubated, no case of Horner syndrome occurred, and one episode of dysphonia occurred requiring no advanced respiratory support.

The bilateral approach described in the present study revealed safe and effective across different subtypes of VT and aetiology of cardiomyopathy.

A case report by Reinertsen et al. [42] describes the effectiveness of PSGB in 13 patients by comparing the number of ventricular arrhythmias and shocks over the 48 and 24 hours before the block and over the 24, 48, 72 and 96 after it. A total of 85% patients received left percutaneous ganglion block with the remaining 15% receiving right percutaneous ganglion block; no bilateral block was performed. All the time intervals between pre- and post-procedure revealed a decrease in arrhythmias and shocks. A total of 54% patients received dexamethasone (4–12 mg) with lidocaine or ropivacaine with an administration volume of 8–20 ml. Transient hypotension was the only adverse event recorded.

In a retrospective study on 18 patients with AS, Sanghai et al. [43] compared the safety and effectiveness of one single injection (SI) versus continuous infusion (CI). CI lasted an average of 2.2 ± 0.9 days after the initial injection. A reduction of 75% arrhythmias was registered at 24 hours after PSGB (CI group vs SI group 94% vs 45%, $p = 0.01$). CI also reported fewer relapses compared with SI (CI 78% vs SI 56%). In the SI group, the procedure was repeated in four cases out of nine (44%) and with an average of 2 days from the first block. In-hospital survival rates were similar between groups with one episode of temporary hyposthenia of the arm and no other complications. The lower number of relapses over the long term in patients with continuous infusion confirms the cardinal role of the sympathetic block in the treatment of AS.

In our case series, a total of 18 PSGB were performed in 11 patients. We conducted two different analyses with a per-patient and a per-procedure approach to avoid an overestimation of PSGB effectiveness in case of repeated procedures. The analysis of the procedures was based on 1-hour intervals to avoid overlapping with the index PSGB and to minimise the effect of the spontaneous reduction of arrhythmias. The study demonstrated VT reduction within 1 h following each PSGB and the complete elimination of arrhythmias in 83% cases. In the per-patient analysis, the average number of VT significantly decreased (7 vs 1, $p = 0.002$) over the 24 hours following multiple procedures. Despite the anatomical approach and no sedation in most cases (14 out of 18 blocks), no adverse event occurred (Table 5.3).

Table 5.3 List of case series on percutaneous stellate ganglion block

Author year	No. of cases	Heart disease	FE	Arrhythmias	Antiarrhythmic drugs used	SGB technique used	Effectiveness	Complications	Conclusion	Notes
Nademanee et al. [36] 2000	**49 pts: Group 1** SNS block (27 pcs): **6/27 PSGB**, (21 with BB); **group 2:** Antiarrhythmic sec ACLS	Recent acute myocardial infarction 28/49 anterior AMI 6/49 inferior 5/49 NSTEMI 10/49 anterior and inferior IMA	32 ± 8%	TV/FV	Esmolol, propranolol, lidocaine, procainamide, bretylium, amiodarone	Anatomical anterior approach, left side only, with lidocaine. Possibly repeatable with lidocaine or magnesium	7-day mortality: Group 1 vs group 2: 82% vs 22% Survival considered at 1-year follow-up: group 1 vs group 2: 67% vs 5%	No	SNS blockade is superior to antiarrhythmic therapy recommended by the ACLS guidelines. SNS blockade patients have better survival at 1 week and 1 year. SNS block should be the treatment of choice in storm versus antiarrhythmic drugs according to ACLS	41/49 under general anaesthesia for 24–48 h after the storm Markers of sympatholysis by PSGB: Complete or partial Horner's syndrome
Amino et al. [37] 2007	15 pts.: **11 pcs with LSGB,** 4 pcs without LSGB	All in refractory cardiac arrest. Structural ischaemic and non-ischaemic heart disease in 11/11	40%	TV/FV	Nifekalant, lidocaine	Left anterior (not stated if anatomical or ultrasound-guided) with lidocaine, bupivacaine, mepivacaine or ropivacaine. Performed after administration of nifekalant in case of failure	Successful defibrillation in 7/11 LSGB vs non-LSGB mortality 45% vs 100%	No	The combination of nifekalant ev with LSGB is useful in the defibrillation of intractable VT/FV and is a strategy for VT/FV resistant to antiarrhythmic Ikr blockers	Nifekalant administered to all patients Markers of sympatholysis by PSGB: Pre- and post-PSGB pupillary diameter

(continued)

Table 5.3 (continued)

Author year	No. of cases	Heart disease	FE	Arrhythmias	Antiarrhythmic drugs used	SGB technique used	Effectiveness	Complications	Conclusion	Notes
Prabhu et al. [38] 2016	9 pts. LSCD of which **5** pts. **PSGB**	Structural ischaemic and non-ischaemic heart disease in 8/9 patients	20–55%	TV/FV	Metoprolol, verapamil, amiodarone, lidocaine	Left anterior ultrasound-guided with bupivacaine on intubated patients	1/5 not effective 1/5 effective 3/5 effectiveness not quantifiable for PSGB+LSCD	No	PSGB is a *salvage procedure* in centres where surgical denervation or transcatheter ablation is not available	Of the two PSGB (not followed by LSCD), one died from arrhythmic storm and one from sudden death 4 days after storm termination. The three PSGB+LSCD patients discharged alive Markers of sympatholysis: Horner's syndrome, increased temperature and anhidrosis
Garcia et al. [39] 2016	8 pts. with PSGB	Structural ischaemic and non-ischaemic heart disease in 7/8 patients	32%	Polymor phic TV	BB, amiodarone, procainamide, lidocaine, magnesium	Left anterior ultrasound-guided with ropivacaine. Continuous infusion is planned.	6/8 LSBG effective in reducing arrhythmias at 24 h 3/8 recurrences at 24 h but >3 days apart	No	LSGB is useful in treating refractory electrical storm	2/8 nonresponders to LSGB received TEA. Infusion duration from 2 to 10 days 4/8 deceased but only 1/8 died of arrhythmic causes Markers of sympatholysis: Horner's syndrome for PSGB and disappearance of chest pain for TEA

Tian et al. [40] 2019	30 pts.: 15 only left 15 bilateral 38 PSGB performed	Structural heart disease in 27/30: Ischaemic 17/30, non-ischaemic 10/30; nonstructural with unstable VT 2/30, LQTS 1/30	34%	TV/FV	At least two antiarrhythmic drugs, amiodarone and lidocaine	Ultrasound-guided direct postero-anterior technique or antero-lateral technique under fluoroscopic guidance. First left then right in case of recurrences. Bilateral block only on intubated patients Bupivacaine (28/38) and/or lidocaine Provision is made for repetition in case of relapse at the end of the effect	Number of TV/FV -72 h vs +72 h 11 (3–163) vs 0 (0–12); $p < 0.001$ 7/30 deaths: 2/7 due to arrhythmias	No	PSGB effective in treating arrhythmic storm without adverse effects. Patients with arrhythmic recurrences are more often non-ischaemic and have a history of ventricular arrhythmias with a longer cycle	70% SGB during general anaesthesia, 30% SGB sedation Marker of sympatholysis: Temperature change

(continued)

Table 5.3 (continued)

Author year	No. of cases	Heart disease	FE	Arrhythmias	Antiarrhythmic drugs used	SGB technique used	Effectiveness	Complications	Conclusion	Notes
Fudim et al. [41] 2020	20 pts. PSGB bilateral	Structural heart disease 10/20 ischaemic 10/20 non-ischaemic	<35% in 16/20	TV/FV	BB, lidocaine, amiodarone, procainamide	Bilateral ultrasound	TV/FV -24 h vs +24 h 4.5 (2–12.8) vs 0 (0–2); $p < 0.001$ Shock −24 h vs +24 h 2 (0–10.3) vs 0 (0–0.8); $p = 0.002$ TV/FV -48 h vs +48 h 5.5 (2–15.8) vs 0 (0–3.8); $p < 0.001$ Shock −48 h vs +48 h 2.5 (0–10.3) vs 0 (0–2.5); $p = 0.002$	1 transient dysphonia	Bilateral PSGB is safe and effective in reducing ventricular arrhythmias and shocks regardless of the type of heart disease and type of arrhythmia	5/20 PSGB repeated with average time of 6 days between first and second injection; 2/20 3 PSGB 9/20 IABP, Impella, LVAD/RVAD, ECMO 7/20 in-hospital death but none from arrhythmic causes No patients showed Horner's syndrome but possible underestimation because 60% Intubated patients
Reinertsen et al. [42] 2021	13 pts., 11/13 left and 2/13 right	Structural heart disease in 13/13	23%	TWA/td P/TV/FV	Amiodarone, lidocaine, quinidine, ranolazine, phenytoin, procainamide	Unilateral ultrasound with lidocaine or bupivacaine and dexamethasone or ropivacaine. Left only in 11/13, right only in 2/13, at the level of C6 in 12/13, at the level of C5 in 1/13	Significant reduction in VT/FV and shocks at 24, 48, 72 and 96 h At 96 h 62% of pts. free of arrhythmias and 92% free of shocks	1 hypotension	PSGB reduces ventricular arrhythmias and defibrillation for up to 96 h	IABP, LVAD, ECMO Dexamethasone in injection to increase the effect of the local anaesthetic Not assessed for Horner's syndrome and dysphonia due to confounding factors such as sedation

Sanghai et al. [43] 2021	18 pts. 9 single injection (SI) 9 continuous infusion (CI)	Structural heart disease in 16/18 (7/18 post-ischaemic, 9/18 non-ischaemic) channelopathy (LQTS) 2/18	30.9 ± 12.1%	13/18 TV 5/18 TV/FV	Amiodarone + lidocaine 11/18 amiodarone 4/18 lidocaine 3/18	Left monolateral ultrasound-guided lateral approach with ropivacaine or bupivacaine	AV/24 h pre-SGB vs post-SGB % recurrence **Overall** 1.6 (0.5–3) vs 0 (0–0.4); $p < 0.001$ 75% reduction in AV compared to baseline 67% free of ventricular arrhythmias **SI Group** 1 (0.3–2.8) vs 0 (0–1); $p = 0.008$ 45% reduction in AV compared to baseline 56% no recidivism **Group CI** 2.5 (1.5–3) vs 0 (0–0) $p = 0.004$ 94% reduction in AV compared to baseline 78% no recurrence	No major upper limb Hyposthenia (1); Dysphonia (1)	SI and CI approaches are effective and safe. Continuous infusion reduces ventricular burden, reduces the need to perform multiple procedures and does not increase acute adverse events or hospital outcome	Sedation, antiarrhythmic drugs and external circulatory support balanced between pre- and post-SGB to avoid overestimating the effectiveness of SGB No sedation/ intubation before performing SGB The pre-SGB period begins after the administration of antiarrhythmic iv so as to isolate the effect of SGB alone Note dysphonia, ptosis and asthenia upper limb

(continued)

Table 5.3 (continued)

Author year	No. of cases	Heart disease	FE	Arrhythmias	Antiarrhythmic drugs used	SGB technique used	Effectiveness	Complications	Conclusion	Notes
Savastano et al. [44]. 2021	11 18 PSGB performed 16 bolo only 2 bolus + infusion	Structural heart disease, ischaemic and non-ischaemic, in 11/11	31.6%	TV/FV	Amiodarone, lidocaine	Anatomical unilateral anterior with lidocaine and/or bupivacaine	Analysis per patient: Shock/ATP -24 h vs +24 h 7 (4.3–12) vs 1 (0–1.8); $p = 0.002$ Analysis by block shock/ATP -1 h vs +1 h 5 (1–10) vs 0 (0–0); $p < 0.001$	No	Anterior anatomical approach is safe and well tolerated, effective in reducing arrhythmic recurrences.	Anisocoria observed in only 5/18 procedures ECMO, IABP 22% procedures done in intubation

IMA acute myocardial infarction, *BB* beta-blockers, *SNS* sympathetic nervous system, *VT* ventricular tachycardia, *VF* ventricular fibrillation, *ACLS* advanced cardiovascular life support, *TEA* thoracic epidural anaesthesia, *PSGB* percutaneous ganglion block, *PSGB* percutaneous ganglion block, *PRSGB* right percutaneous ganglion block, *ATP* antitachycardia pacing, *LQTS* long QT syndrome

Multicentre Studies

Two multicentre trials on PSGB as a treatment for ventricular arrhythmias refractory to conventional therapy were published in 2024.

Chouairi et al. presented [45] the analysis from a multicentre registry of patients treated with PSGB for refractory ventricular arrhythmia between 2016 and 2022 at the Institute for Clinical and Experimental Medicine (IKEM) in the Czech Republic and the Duke University School of Medicine, North Carolina, USA. A total of 117 patients with refractory ventricular arrhythmias underwent ultrasound-guided PSGB, with 24 of these receiving bilateral PSGB. By comparing the 24 h before and after PSGB, the study demonstrated a significant reduction in the median episodes of VT/VF (7.5 vs 1.0, $p < 0.001$) and a significant reduction in the median defibrillation events (2.0 vs 0.0, $p < 0.001$). Two complications occurred in the Duke patient cohort: one patient experienced hoarseness due to recurrent laryngeal nerve block and another patient had brachial plexus block. Both the complications resolved within 1 day without further intervention.

Our multicentre observational STAR [46] study enrolled patients with electrical storm refractory to standard treatment from July 1, 2017, to June 30, 2023. A total of 131 patients from 19 centres were enrolled and underwent 184 PSGBs. STAR operators were specifically trained in both the anterior anatomical and the lateral ultrasound-guided approaches. The primary outcome, a reduction of treated arrhythmic events by at least 50% comparing the 12 h following PSGB with the 12 h before the procedure, was achieved in 92% of patients, and the median reduction in arrhythmic episodes between 12 h before and after PSGB was 100% (IR −100% to −92.3%). Arrhythmic episodes requiring treatment were significantly reduced comparing 12 h before the first PSGB with 12 h after the last procedure (6 vs 0, $p < 0.0001$), as well as comparing 1 h before with 1 h after each procedure (2 vs 0, $p < 0.001$), demonstrating a significant reduction of the number of ATP/shocks both on a per-patient and per-procedure analysis. The other primary outcome was the safety of the technique: only one major complication occurred due to systemic lidocaine absorption in a patient who was also receiving an intravenous lidocaine infusion, which was rapidly resolved with lipid infusion. These results confirmed that PSGB is a safe and effective technique for treating refractory electrical storm and should be considered to stabilise patients unresponsive to first-line conventional treatments.

The secondary outcomes clarified several aspects: (1) PSGB demonstrated similar efficacy regardless of the presence of anisocoria, (2) both the anatomical and ultrasound-guided approaches showed significant reduction in treated arrhythmias, (3) both bolus and continuous infusion methods exhibited similar and significant efficacy, and (4) centres with low and high patient enrolment volumes demonstrated comparable efficacy, highlighting that a relatively simple training may be sufficient suggesting that this approach is generalisable on a large scale (Table 5.4).

Table 5.4 Multicentre studies on percutaneous stelate ganglion block

Author year	No. of cases	Heart disease	FE	Arrhythmias	Antiarrhythmic drugs used	SGB technique used	Effectiveness	Complications	Conclusion	Notes
Chouairi et al. [45] 2024	2 centres 117 pts	Structural heart disease, ischaemic and non-ischaemic	27%	TV/FV	Amiodarone, lidocaine, procainamide, mexiletine, quinidine	Ultrasound-guided approach Left side if unilateral PSGB 21/117 bilateral PSGB Bupivacaine, ropivacaine, lidocaine	Median episodes of VT/VF -24 h vs +24 h: 7.5 (3.0–27.0) vs 1.0 (0.0–4.5), $p < 0.001$ Median defibrilla-tion -24 h vs +24 h: 2.0 (0.0–8.0) vs 0.0 (0.0–1.0), $p < 0.001$	2 complications (1 recurrent laryngeal nerve block resulting in hoarseness and 1 brachial plexus block), both resolved within 1 day	PSGB is associated with a reduction in the VT/VF burden and need for defibrillation	Both unilateral and bilateral PSGBs are associated with a reduced burden of VT/VF
Savastano et al. [46] 2024	19 centres 131 pts. 184 PSGBs performed	Structural heart disease, ischaemic and non-ischaemic, channelopathies 27/131 cardiogenic shock, 7/131 septic shock, 11/131 cardiac arrest	25%	TV/FV	Amiodarone, lidocaine, procainamide, beta-blockers	106/184 anatomical approach, 78/184 ultrasound-guided approach 152/184 bolus only, 32/184 bolus + infusion 181/184 left, 3/184 right Lidocaine, bupivacaine, ropivacaine, mepivacaine	92% of patients showed a reduction of ATP/shock >50% in the 12 h after PSGB Per-patient analysis: Shock/ATP -12 h vs +12 h 6 (3–15.8) vs 0 (0–1), $p < 0.001$ Per-procedure analysis shock/ATP -1 h vs +1 h 2 (0–6) vs 0 (0–0); $p < 0.0001$	1 major complication due to systemic lidocaine absorption, rapidly resolved with lipid infusion	PSGB is a safe and effective technique to treat refractory electrical storm and should be considered to stabilise patients unresponsive to First-line conventional treatments	Efficacy regardless of the appearance of anisocoria Significant reduction of treated arrhythmias with both anatomical and ultrasound-guided approach Similar and significant efficacy with both methods (bolus and continuous infusion) Similar efficacy in low- and high-enrolment volume centres

Final Considerations

The abovementioned body of evidence depicts percutaneous stellate ganglion block as a safe and effective technique.

PSGB has been mentioned in some treatment algorithms for managing electrical storm since 2015. Sorajja et al. [47] reported PSGB as a potential treatment for polymorphic ventricular tachycardia, with or without myocardial ischaemia, or for ventricular fibrillation, exclusively during ischaemia (Fig. 5.1).

However, the cases described above confirmed that PSGB can be considered also for monomorphic tachycardia and for LQTS as well. In a more recent therapeutic algorithm by Kowlgi [48], PSGB is mentioned as a viable option in case of haemodynamically stable VT. PSGB can be effectively performed in case of instable VT and in case of cardiac arrest, including those requiring ECMO, across both adult and paediatric patients (Fig. 5.2).

For the first time, the European Society of Cardiology (ESC) in 2022 [49] considered neuromodulation with a class IIB indication for electrical storm management in case of polymorphic TV in patients with LQTS or CPVT and in case of monomorphic VT after a series of treatment have failed such as sedation, antiarrhythmic drugs and ablation. Similar indications have come in 2024 also from a consensus by the European Heart Rhythm Association (EHRA) [50] and probably may be extended [51], also considering that these recommendations have been issued before the publications of the two large multicentric studies on this technique. Furthermore, guidelines' indications are referred to neuromodulation which

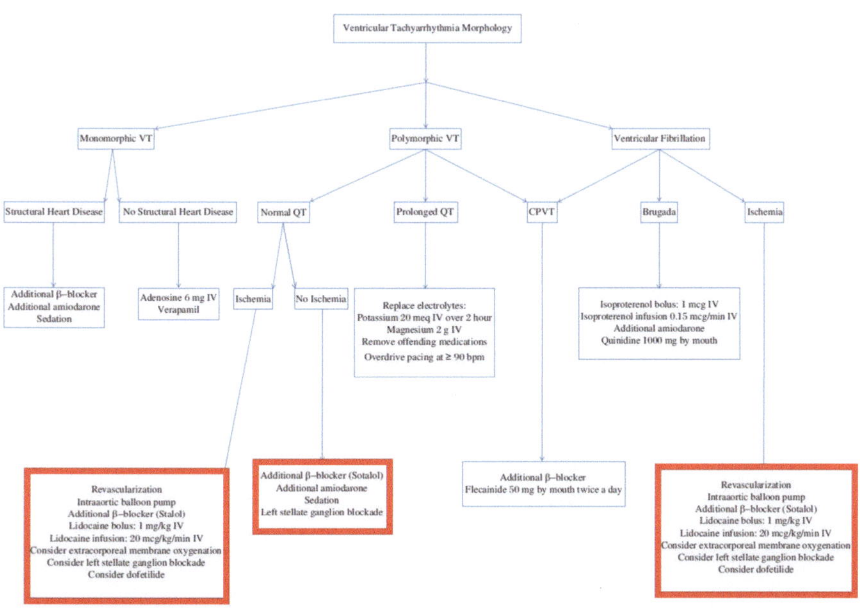

Fig. 5.1 Algorithm of treatment of the electrical storm. In red: cells where PSGB in an option. (Modified from the work by Sorajja et al. [47])

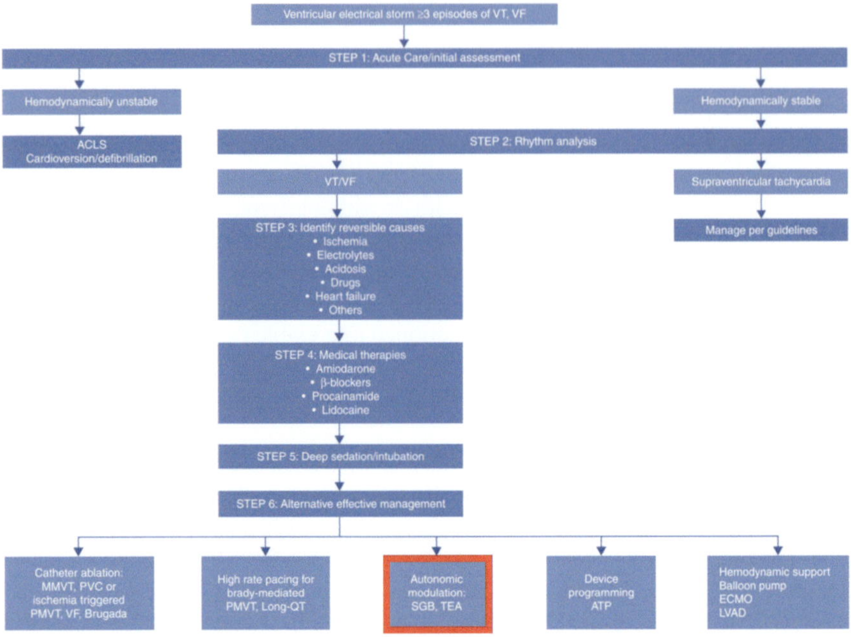

Fig. 5.2 Algorithm for the treatment of patients with electrical storm (AS). (Modified from Kowlgi et al. [48])

encompasses three different procedures: surgical sympathetic denervation, stellate ganglion block and thoracic epidural anaesthesia (TEA). These techniques differ in many aspects, require different training and equipment and have different contraindications [52]. Notably, PSGB is easier, versatile and with fewer contraindications.

Currently, albeit some data suggest that slower ventricular tachycardia may be less responsive to the procedure, criteria to establish the ideal candidate to PSGB, optimal timing to perform it or the safest and most effective technique have yet not been defined. Owing to these limitations and to the absence of multicentric randomised studies, we can conclude that PSGB can be safely used in the vast majority of cases of electrical storm.

References

1. Schwartz PJ, Snebold NG, Brown AM. Effects of unilateral cardiac sympathetic denervation on the ventricular fibrillation threshold. Am J Cardiol. 1976;37(7):1034–40. https://doi.org/10.1016/0002-9149(76)90420-3.
2. Casati R, Lombardi F, Malliani A. Afferent sympathetic unmyelinated fibres with left ventricular endings in cats. J Physiol. 1979;292:135–48. https://doi.org/10.1113/jphysiol.1979.sp012842. PMID: 490336; PMCID: PMC1280849.
3. Grossman MA. Cardiac arrhythmias in acute central nervous system disease: successful management with stellate ganglion block. Arch Intern Med. 1976;136(2):203–7. https://doi.org/10.1001/archinte.1976.03630020057012.

4. Burch GE, Meyers R, Abildskov JA. A new electrocardiographic pattern observed in cerebrovascular accidents. Circulation. 1954;9(5):719–23. https://doi.org/10.1161/01.CIR.9.5.719.
5. Moss AJ, McDonald J. Unilateral cervicothoracic sympathetic ganglionectomy for the treatment of long QT interval syndrome. N Engl J Med. 1971;285(16):903–4. https://doi.org/10.1056/nejm197110142851607.
6. Biagini A, Sabino F, Paladini G, Severi S, Marraccini P, Contini C, L'Abbate A. Treatment of perinfarction recurrent ventricular fibrillation by percutaneous pharmacological block of left stellate ganglion. Clin Cardiol. 1985;8(2):111–3. https://doi.org/10.1002/clc.4960080209. PMID: 3971606.
7. Hoepp HW, Eggeling T, Hombach V. Pharmacologic blockade of the left stellate ganglion using a drug-reservoir-pump system. Chest. 1990;97(1):250–1. https://doi.org/10.1378/chest.97.1.250.
8. Patel RA, Priore DL, Szeto WY, Slevin KA. Left stellate ganglion blockade for the management of drug-resistant electrical storm. Pain Med. 2011;12(8):1196–8. https://doi.org/10.1111/J.1526-4637.2011.01167.X.
9. Loyalka P, Hariharan R, Gholkar G, et al. Left stellate ganglion block for continuous ventricular arrhythmias during percutaneous left ventricular assist device support. Tex Heart Inst J. 2011;38(4):409–11.
10. Tan AY, Abdi S, Buxton AE, Anter E. Percutaneous stellate ganglia block for acute control of refractory ventricular tachycardia. Heart Rhythm. 2012;9(12):2063–7. https://doi.org/10.1016/J.HRTHM.2012.07.030.
11. Hayase J, Patel J, Narayan SM, Krummen DE. Percutaneous stellate ganglion block suppressing VT and VF in a patient refractory to VT ablation. J Cardiovasc Electrophysiol. 2013;24(8):926–8.
12. García-Morán E, Sandín-Fuentes MG, Álvarez López JC, Duro-Aguado I, Urueña-Martínez N, Hernández-Luis C. Tormenta arrítmica secundaria a infarto agudo de miocardio e insuficiencia cardiaca tratada mediante bloqueo de ganglio estrellado izquierdo. Rev Esp Cardiol. 2013;66(7):595–7. https://doi.org/10.1016/j.recesp.2013.01.016.
13. Gadhinglajkar S, Sreedhar R, Unnikrishnan M, Namboodiri N. Electrical storm: role of stellate ganglion blockade and anesthetic implications of left cardiac sympathetic denervation. Indian J Anaesth. 2013;57(4):397–400. https://doi.org/10.4103/0019-5049.118568.
14. Mata Francisco NC, Gómez Pesquera E, Ruiz López N, Álvarez López JC, Jorge-Monjas P. Tratamiento de las arritmias cardíacas refractarias mediante bloqueo del ganglio estrellado en un paciente. Acceso por técnica clásica y ecodirigida. Rev Esp Anestesiol Reanim. 2014;61(8):454–6. https://doi.org/10.1016/j.redar.2013.08.007.
15. Malik AA, Khan AA, Dingmann K, et al. Percutaneous inferior cervical sympathetic ganglion blockade for the treatment of ventricular tachycardia storm: case report and review of the literature. J Vasc Interv Neurol. 2014;7(5):48. /pmc/articles/PMC4280879/. Accessed December 26, 2021
16. Hulata DF, Le-Wendling L, Boezaart AP, Hurley RW. Stellate ganglion local anesthetic blockade and neurolysis for the treatment of refractory ventricular fibrillation. A A Case Rep. 2015;4(5):49–51. https://doi.org/10.1213/XAA.0000000000000124.
17. Scanlon MM, Gillespie SM, Schaff HV, Cha YM, Wittwer ED. Urgent ultrasound-guided bilateral stellate ganglion blocks in a patient with medically refractory ventricular arrhythmias. Crit Care Med. 2015;43(8):e316–8. https://doi.org/10.1097/CCM.0000000000001086.
18. Smith DI, Jones C, Morris GK, Kralovic S, Massey HT, Sifain A. Trial ultrasound-guided continuous left stellate ganglion blockade before surgical gangliolysis in a patient with a left ventricular assist device and intractable ventricular tachycardia: a pain control application to a complex hemodynamic condition. ASAIO J. 2015;61(1):104–6. https://doi.org/10.1097/MAT.0000000000000163.
19. Fudim M, Boortz-Marx R, Patel CB, Sun AY, Piccini JP. Autonomic modulation for the treatment of ventricular arrhythmias: therapeutic use of percutaneous stellate ganglion blocks. J Cardiovasc Electrophysiol. 2017;28(4):446–9. https://doi.org/10.1111/jce.13152.

20. Przybylski A, Romanek J, Chlebuś M, Deręgowska B, Kuzniar J. Percutaneous stellate ganglion block as an adjunctive therapy in the treatment of incessant ventricular tachycardia. Kardiol Pol. 2018;76(6):1018–20. https://doi.org/10.5603/KP.2018.0120.
21. Yang SC, Wu CC, Hsieh YJ. Left stellate ganglion block, a rescue treatment for ventricular arrhythmia refractory to radiofrequency catheter ablation: a care-compliant case report. Medicine (Baltimore). 2019;98(44):e17790. https://doi.org/10.1097/MD.0000000000017790.
22. Savastano S, Pugliese L, Baldi E, Dusi V, Tavazzi G, De Ferrari GM. Percutaneous continuous left stellate ganglion block as an effective bridge to bilateral cardiac sympathetic denervation. Europace. 2020;22(4):606. https://doi.org/10.1093/EUROPACE/EUAA007.
23. Savastano S, Baldi E, Camporotondo R, Belliato M, Marinoni B, De Ferrari GM. Percutaneous stellate ganglion block and extracorporeal cardiopulmonary resuscitation: an effective and safe combination for refractory ventricular fibrillation. Europace. 2020;22(1):148. https://doi.org/10.1093/EUROPACE/EUZ180.
24. Sahoo R, Kar R, Dev I, Kumar M, Parida A, Ganguly A. Stellate ganglion block as rescue therapy in drug-resistant electrical storm. Ann Card Anaesth. 2021;24(3):415. https://doi.org/10.4103/ACA.ACA_168_19.
25. Pillai A, Koneru JN, Ellenbogen KA, Padala SK. Case Report Clinical Case Autonomic modulation for treatment of repolarization alternans and refractory ventricular electrical storm. 2021. doi:https://doi.org/10.1016/j.jaccas.2021.06.040.
26. Mohd Y, Kumar A, Sheikh I, et al. Calming the storm—stellate ganglion block in refractory ventricular arrhythmia in the emergency department. Am J Emerg Med. 2021;45(December):685.e5–8. https://doi.org/10.1016/j.ajem.2020.12.063.
27. Ajijola OA, Lellouche N, Bourke T, et al. Bilateral cardiac sympathetic denervation for the management of electrical storm. J Am Coll Cardiol. 2012;59(1):91–2. https://doi.org/10.1016/j.jacc.2011.09.043.
28. Jervell A, Lange-Nielsen F. Congenital deaf-mutism, functional heart disease with prolongation of the Q-T interval, and sudden death. Am Heart J. 1957;54(1):59–68. https://doi.org/10.1016/0002-8703(57)90079-0.
29. Romano C, Gemme GRP. Rare cardiac arrythmias of the pediatric age. II. Syncopal attacks due to paroxysmal ventricular fibrillation. (presentation of 1st case in Italian pediatric literature). Clin Pediatr. 1963;45:656.
30. Ward OC. A new familial cardiac syndrome in children. J Irish Med Assoc. 1964;54:103–6. https://europepmc.org/article/med/14136838. Accessed February 2, 2022
31. Yanagida H, Kemi C, Suwa K. The effects of stellate ganglion block on the idiopathic prolongation of the Q-T interval with cardiac arrhythmia (The Romano Ward syndrome). Anesth Analg. 1976;55(6):782–7. https://doi.org/10.1213/00000539-197611000-00007.
32. Parris WCV, Reddy BC, White HW, McGrath DM. Stellate ganglion blocks in pediatric patients. Anesth Analg. 1991;72(4):552–6. https://doi.org/10.1213/00000539-199104000-00024.
33. Mesa A, Kaplan RF. Dysrhythmias controlled with stellate ganglion block in a child with diabetes and a variant of long QT syndrome. Reg Anesth. 1993;18(1):60–2.
34. Franklin AD, Llobet JR, Sobey CM, Daniels JM, Kannankeril PJ. Stellate ganglion catheter effective for treatment of ventricular tachycardia storm in a pediatric patient on extracorporeal membrane oxygenation: a case report. A&A Pract. 2019;13(7):245–9. https://doi.org/10.1213/XAA.0000000000001036.
35. Boe BA, Webster G, Asher Y, Tsao S, Suresh S, Steinhorn DM. Percutaneous, ultrasound-guided stellate ganglion nerve block suppresses recurrent ventricular fibrillation in an infant awaiting heart transplant. Circ Arrhythm Electrophysiol. 2012;5(5):93–4. https://doi.org/10.1161/CIRCEP.112.974329.
36. Nademanee K, Taylor R, Bailey WE, Rieders DE, Kosar EM. Treating electrical storm: sympathetic blockade versus advanced cardiac life support-guided therapy. Circulation. 2000;102(7):742–7. https://doi.org/10.1161/01.CIR.102.7.742/FORMAT/EPUB.
37. Amino M, Yoshioka K, Morita S, et al. Is the combination therapy of IKr-channel blocker and left stellate ganglion block effective for intractable ventricular arrhythmia in a cardiopulmonary arrest patient? Cardiol J. 2007;14(4):355–65.

38. Prabhu MA, Prasad SBV, Abhilash SP, Thajudeen A, Balasubramoniam KR, Namboodiri N. Left sympathetic cardiac denervation in managing electrical storm: acute outcome and long term follow up. J Interv Card Electrophysiol. 2016;47(3):285–92. https://doi.org/10.1007/S10840-016-0153-2/TABLES/3.
39. García-Morán E, Sliwinski-Herrera F, Cortes-Villar C, Sandín-Fuentes M, Pastor Báez G, San Román A. Refractory electrical storm: a role for transient sympathetic blockade. Rev Española Cardiol (English Ed). 2016;69(1):76–8. https://doi.org/10.1016/j.rec.2015.08.024.
40. Tian Y, Wittwer ED, Kapa S, et al. Effective use of percutaneous stellate ganglion blockade in patients with electrical storm. Circ Arrhythm Electrophysiol. 2019;12:9. https://doi.org/10.1161/CIRCEP.118.007118.
41. Fudim M, Qadri YJ, Waldron NH, et al. Stellate ganglion blockade for the treatment of refractory ventricular arrhythmias. JACC Clin Electrophysiol. 2020;6(5):562–71. https://doi.org/10.1016/j.jacep.2019.12.017.
42. Reinertsen E, Sabayon M, Riso M, Lloyd M, Spektor B. Stellate ganglion blockade for treating refractory electrical storm: a historical cohort study Bloc du ganglion stellaire pour le traitement des tempêtes e ́lectriques réfractaires : une e ́tude de cohorte historique. Can J Anesth Can d'anesthésie. 2021:68. https://doi.org/10.1007/s12630.
43. Sanghai S, Abbott NJ, Dewland TA, et al. Stellate ganglion blockade with continuous infusion versus single injection for treatment of ventricular arrhythmia storm. JACC Clin Electrophysiol. 2021;7(4):452–60. https://doi.org/10.1016/j.jacep.2020.09.032.
44. Savastano S, Dusi V, Baldi E, et al. Anatomical-based percutaneous left stellate ganglion block in patients with drug-refractory electrical storm and structural heart disease: a single-Centre case series. Europace. 2021;23(4):581–6. https://doi.org/10.1093/europace/euaa319.
45. Chouairi F, Rajkumar K, Benak A, Qadri Y, Piccini JP, Mathew J, Ray ND, Toman J, Kautzner J, Ganesh A, Sramko M, Fudim M. A multicenter study of stellate ganglion block as a temporizing treatment for refractory ventricular arrhythmias. JACC Clin Electrophysiol. 2024;10(4):750–8.
46. Savastano S, Baldi E, Compagnoni S, Rordorf R, Sanzo A, Gentile FR, Dusi V, Frea S, Gravinese C, Cauti FM, Iannopollo G, De Sensi F, Gandolfi E, Frigerio L, Crea P, Zagari D, Casula M, Sangiorgi G, Persampieri S, Dell'Era G, Patti G, Colombo C, Mugnai G, Notaristefano F, Barengo A, Falcetti R, Perego GB, D'Angelo G, Tanese N, Currao A, Sgromo V, De Ferrari GM, STAR Study Group. Electrical storm treatment by percutaneous stellate ganglion block: the STAR study. Eur Heart J. 2024;45(10):823–33.
47. Sorajja D, Munger TM, Shen WK. Optimal antiarrhythmic drug therapy for electrical storm. J Biomed Res. 2015;29(1):20–34. https://doi.org/10.7555/JBR.29.20140147.
48. Kowlgi GN, Cha YM. Management of ventricular electrical storm: a contemporary appraisal. Europace. 2020;22(12):1768–80. https://doi.org/10.1093/europace/euaa232.
49. Zeppenfeld K, Tfelt-Hansen J, de Riva M, Winkel BG, Behr ER, Blom NA, Charron P, Corrado D, Dagres N, de Chillou C, Eckardt L, Friede T, Haugaa KH, Hocini M, Lambiase PD, Marijon E, Merino JL, Peichl P, Priori SG, Reichlin T, Schulz-Menger J, Sticherling C, Tzeis S, Verstrael A, Volterrani M, ESC Scientific Document Group. 2022 ESC Guidelines for the management of patients with ventricular arrhythmias and the prevention of sudden cardiac death. Eur Heart J. 2022;43(40):3997–4126.
50. Lenarczyk R, Zeppenfeld K, Tfelt-Hansen J, Heinzel FR, Deneke T, Ene E, Meyer C, Wilde A, Arbelo E, Jędrzejczyk-Patej E, Sabbag A, Stühlinger M, di Biase L, Vaseghi M, Ziv O, Bautista-Vargas WF, Kumar S, Namboodiri N, Henz BD, Montero-Cabezas J, Dagres N, Peichl P, Frontera A, Tzeis S, Merino JL, Soejima K, de Chillou C, Tung R, Eckardt L, Maury P, Hlivak P, Tereshchenko LG, Kojodjojo P, Atié J. Management of patients with an electrical storm or clustered ventricular arrhythmias: a clinical consensus statement of the European Heart Rhythm Association of the ESC-endorsed by the Asia-Pacific Heart Rhythm Society, Heart Rhythm Society, and Latin-American Heart Rhythm Society. Europace. 2024;26(4):euae049.
51. Savastano S, Schwartz PJ. Blocking nerves and saving lives: left stellate ganglion block for electrical storms. Heart Rhythm. 2023;20(7):1039–47.
52. Dusi V, Vaseghi M. Neuronal sympathetic block for ventricular arrhythmias: one size may not fit all. Europace. 2023;25(11):euad314.

Part III

How to Perform the Procedure

Anatomy of the Neck

6

Alessandra Palo, Enrico Contri, and Vito Sgromo

The neck is bounded superiorly by the lower margin of the mandible and posteriorly by a line passing through the angle of the mandible—the mastoid process—and going to the external occipital protuberance. Inferiorly, it is bounded anteriorly by the two clavicles and the jugular incisura, posteriorly by the seventh cervical vertebra (C7), and laterally by the acromion. It is possible to distinguish three anatomical regions:

- Anterior region (supra and subhyoid).
- Lateral region (latero-cervical and supra-clavicular).
- Nuchal region.

Anterior Region

Supra-Hyoid

Bounded superiorly by the inferior mandibular margin and inferiorly by the hyoid bone, its lateral boundary is the anterior margin of the sternocleidomastoid muscles. This area is not rich in structures and consists mainly in the muscles of the floor of the mouth (hyoglossus, stylohyoid, mylohyoid, digastric), submandibular and submandibular lymph nodes, and salivary glands.

(translated by Chiara Barbaglia)

A. Palo · E. Contri · V. Sgromo (✉)
Fondazione IRCCS Policlinico San Matteo, Pavia, Italy

AREU Lombardia, AAT 118, Pavia, Italy
e-mail: v.sgromo@smatteo.pv.it

S. Savastano (ed.), *Percutaneous Stellate Ganglion Block for Electrical Storm*,
https://doi.org/10.1007/978-3-031-81762-5_6

Subhyoid (Fig. 6.1)

This region is bounded superiorly by a line passing through the hyoid bone, laterally by the anterior margin of the sternocleidomastoid muscles and inferiorly by the jugular incisura of the sternum. Superficially, the thyroid cartilage is visible with the cricoid cartilage and, more caudally, the first tracheal rings. The thyroid cartilage is a shield-shaped structure consisting of two quadrilateral laminae that join at the anterior margin to form the laryngeal prominence or *Adam's apple*. It is connected to the hyoid bone through the thyroid membrane and the median thyroid ligament. Inferiorly, it is connected with the cricoid cartilage through the anterior cricoid ligament. The thyroid and cricoid cartilages, together with the arytenoids, form the supporting structure of the larynx.

The muscular apparatus of the larynx is divided into extrinsic and intrinsic muscles, the latter additionally divided into respiratory and phonatory.

The lobes of the thyroid gland are connected to the sides of the larynx and to the first tracheal rings, and they relate to the right and the left vascular bundles through the peri-thyroid sheath, a dependency of the middle cervical fascia. The sheath delimits the space of the thyroid gland and the vascular bed, interposed between the posterior face of the sheath and of the gland and the parathyroids.

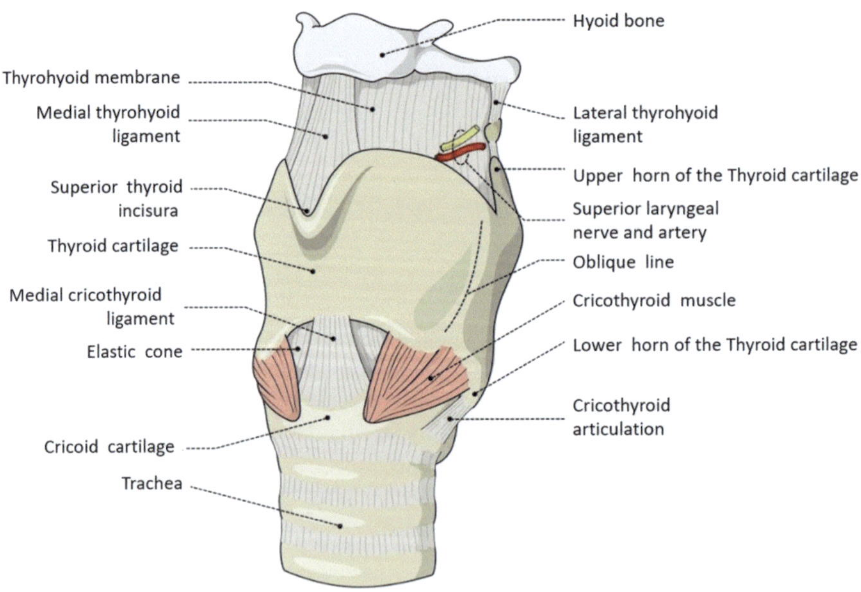

Fig. 6.1 Structure of the larynx, hyoid bone, and first tracheal rings. (Modified by Olek Remesz, figure published under CCBY-SA 2.5)

Lateral Region

Latero-Cervical (Fig. 6.2)

It consists essentially in the sternocleidomastoid muscle, limited at the top by the angle of the mandible and the mastoid process and at the bottom by the middle third of the clavicle and the sternoclavicular joint.

This region includes the neck vascular bundle, which contains the common carotid artery, the internal jugular vein, and the vagus nerve. Within the bundle, the vagus nerve is located most posteriorly, the carotid artery anteriorly and medially to the nerve, and the jugular anterolaterally to the nerve. The structures are wrapped by an aponeurotic fascia derived from the middle cervical fascia.

Supra-Clavicular

This region is limited inferiorly by the clavicle, anteriorly by the posterior margin of the sternocleidomastoid muscle and posteriorly by the trapezius muscle. In depth, this region contracts with the pleural dome, the first rib, and the transverse processes of the cervical vertebrae.

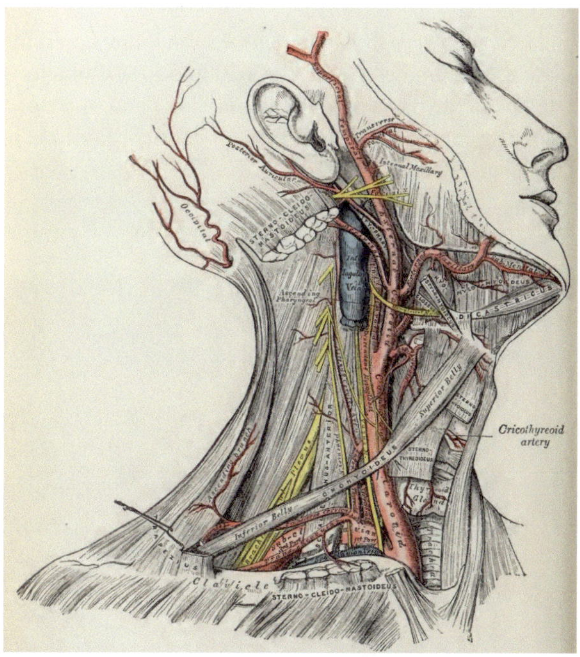

Fig. 6.2 Vascular bundle of the neck, excision of the sternocleidomastoid muscle, and partial resection of the jugular vein. (From Anatomy of the Human Body (Fig. 507). H. Gray. 1918)

Nuchal Region

This region has a triangular shape: at the basis, the line connecting the seventh cervical vertebra to the acromion; at the apex, the external occipital protuberance; and at the sides of the triangle, the two posterior margins of the trapezius muscle.

The anatomical division described above and a deep knowledge of the anatomy of the anterior and lateral regions are essential for a proper execution of the stellate ganglion block by anatomical approach.

The division by cervical bands described below should instead be the basis for performance of the procedure by ultrasound-guided approach (Fig. 6.3).

The *superficial cervical fascia is* located immediately below the skin, the subcutaneous tissue, and platysma muscle—a vast, symmetrical laminar muscle originating at level of the second rib and of the anterior surface of the shoulder, ascending the lateral region of the neck and terminating at level of the masseter region, chin, and labial commissure. The superficial fascia envelops the entire neck; from the anterior midline (cervical linea alba), it runs laterally, wrapping the sternocleidomastoid muscles, and then, posteriorly, the trapezius muscle.

The *middle cervical fascia* is a lamina stretched between the two omohyoid muscles and bordered vertically by the manubrium of the sternum, inferiorly, and by the hyoid bone, superiorly. It contains the thyroid gland, the larynx, and the trachea and gives rise to the aponeurotic fascia that surrounds and delimits the vascular bundle of the neck.

The *deep cervical fascia* delimits the longus colli muscle and other pre-vertebral muscles, the bodies of the cervical and first thoracic vertebrae. Vertically, it originates from the basis of the occipital bone and, inferiorly, it opens into the mediastinum. The inner margin of the deep cervical fascia is in close relationship with the stellate ganglion.

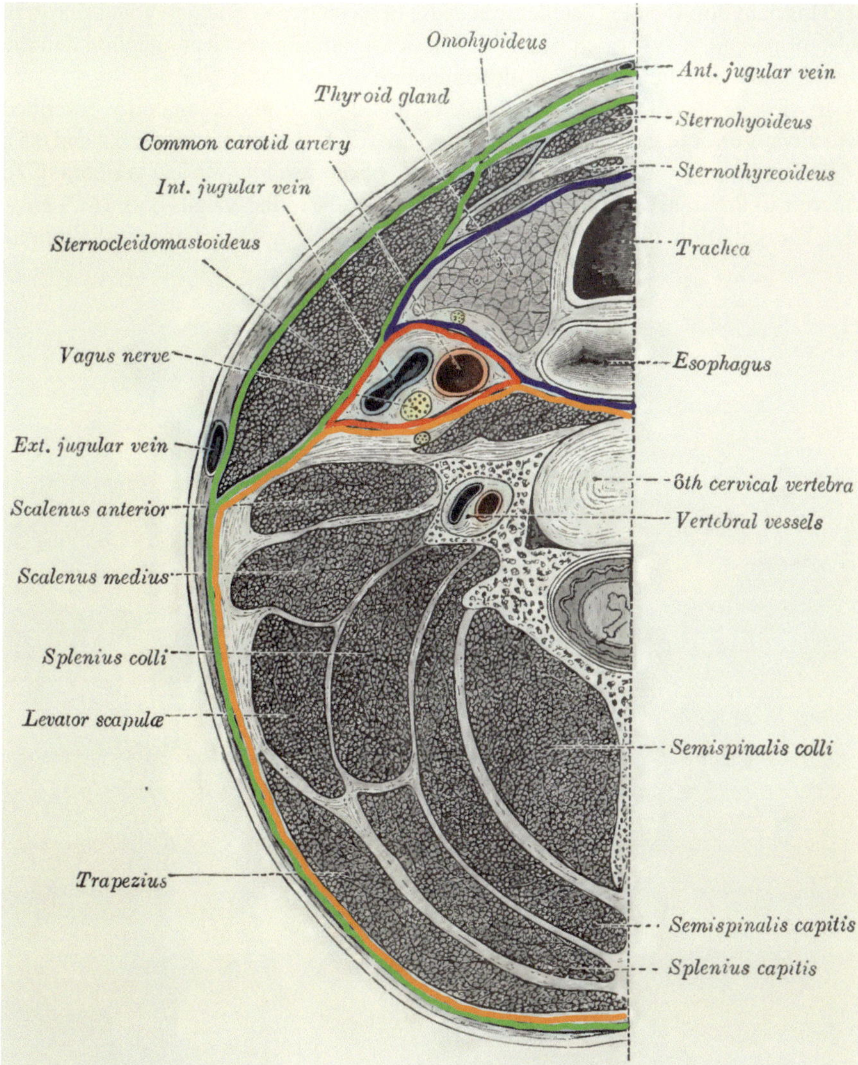

Fig. 6.3 Superficial cervical fascia (green), middle cervical fascia (blue), deep cervical fascia (yellow), and aponeurosis of the neck vascular bundle (red). (Modified from Anatomy of the Human Body (Fig. 384). *H. Gray. 1918*)

The Stellate Ganglion

The stellate ganglion is part of the sympathetic chain, a nerve cord that runs symmetrically down each side of the spinal column, extending from the skull to the coccygeal region, divided into cervical, thoracic, and lumbar regions.

This ganglion is called "stellate" because of its characteristic polygonal shape; in 80% of people, it is formed by the fusion of the inferior cervical ganglion and the first thoracic ganglion, hence the denomination of cervicothoracic.

In view of the therapeutic objective of this discussion, the anatomy described will always refer to the left side of the sympathetic bilateral chain (Figs. 6.4 and 6.5).

The stellate ganglion is located at the level of the seventh cervical vertebra (C7), anterior to the transverse process and anterolaterally to the longus colli (LC) muscle. The ganglion is covered anteriorly by the deep fascia of the neck (lamina

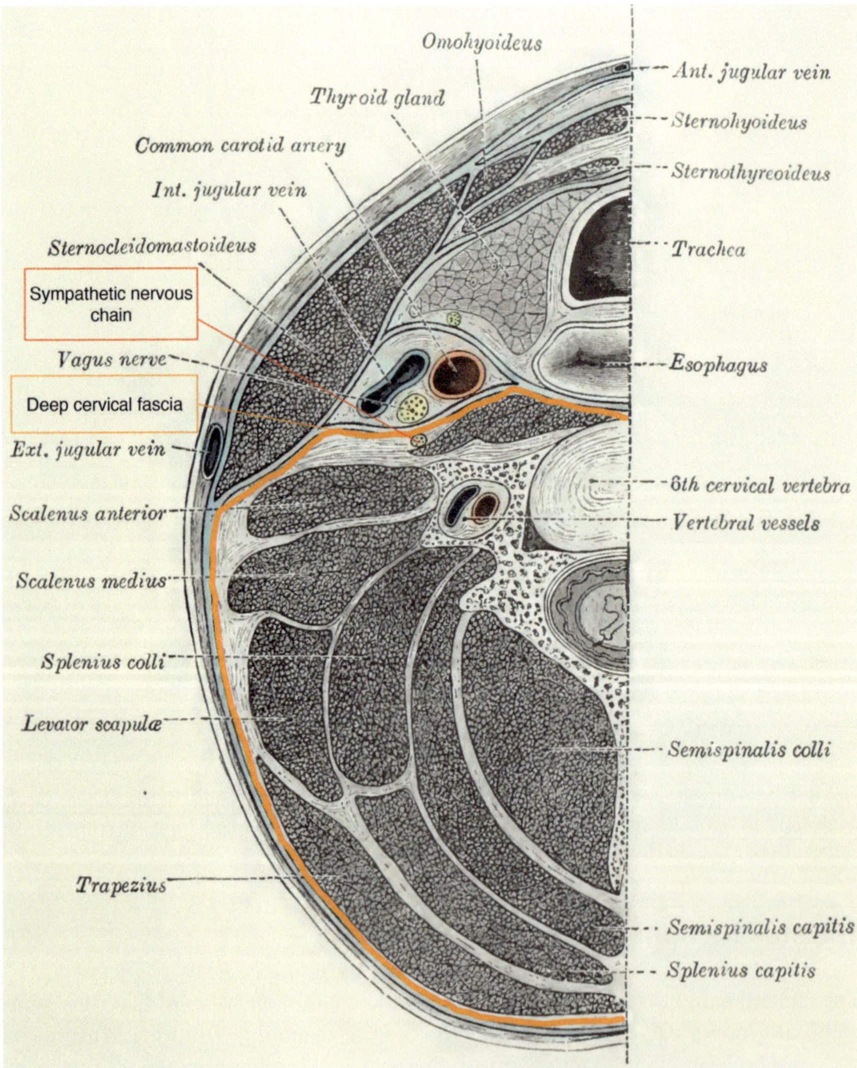

Fig. 6.4 Modified from Anatomy of the Human Body (Fig. 384). H. Gray. 1918

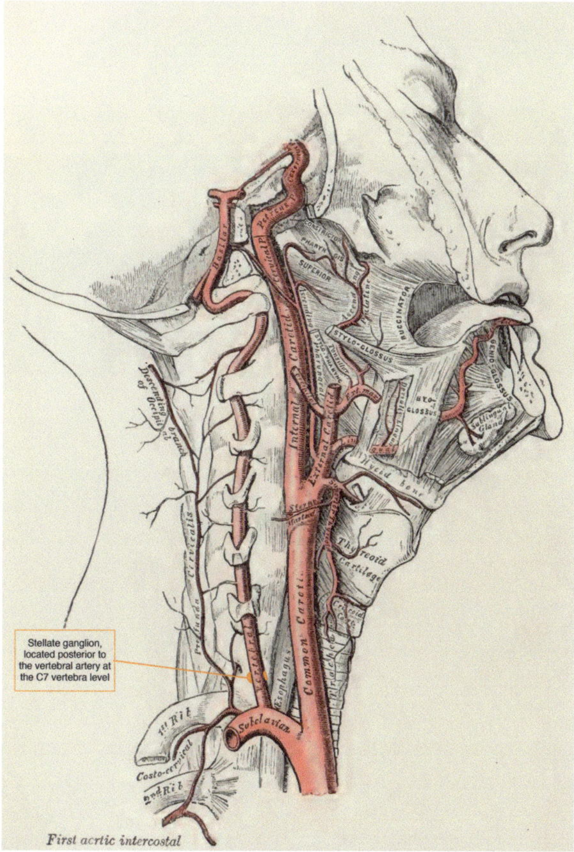

Fig. 6.5 Modified from Anatomy of the Human Body (Fig. 513). H. Gray. 1918

pre-vertebralis). Its position is quite complex: inferiorly, it is located immediately above the subclavian and behind the emergence of the vertebral artery and surrounded by important and delicate structures: the pleural dome inferiorly, the neck vascular bundle (common carotid artery, internal jugular vein, and vagus nerve) anterolaterally, the oesophagus medially, and the thyroid gland, with the inferior thyroid vessels and the recurrent nerve, anteromedially.

Regardless of the technique, an approach at the level of C7 would be complex, as well as burdened by the risk of complications. To limit the risks, the injection of local anaesthetics should be performed at the level of the VI cervical vertebra (C6): here, the region for injection is larger, the vertebral artery has already entered the transverse foramen, and the risk of pneumothorax or subclavian artery puncture is greatly reduced.

If the proper amount of the anaesthetic is correctly injected beyond the pre-vertebral fascia, it will primarily reach the middle cervical ganglion and rapidly spread to the stellate ganglion, without leaking along the vasculo-nervous bundle; this will significantly reduce the risk of a temporary blockage of the outlying nerves and structures (phrenic, recurrent, etc.).

Anterior Approach Using Anatomical Landmarks

7

Simone Savastano and Enrico Baldi

The anatomy of the stellate ganglion is well known and has been described since the nineteenth century. One of its most famous representation was made by Jean-Baptiste Léveillé on anatomical preparation by Ludwik Hirschfeld (Fig. 7.1).

As represented in Fig. 7.1, the stellate ganglion draws its name from its star-like, branching shape derived by the intersection of the last cervical and first thoracic ganglion. It measures 2.5 × 0.5 cm but is generally bigger in males and on the left side. It can have many different shapes and many different connections with the vertebral artery, that, in some cases, can even intersect it [1]. It lies on the longus colli muscle just caudally with respect to the transverse process of vertebra C7. The knowledge of its position is basic to the understanding of the different kinds of block techniques.

Studies on the techniques of the stellate ganglion block for anaesthetic purpose started at the beginning of the twentieth century developing three anatomical approaches [2]:

1. Posterior
2. Antero-lateral
3. Anterior

Labat in 1930, and later White in 1940 [3], respectively, developed and improved the first ganglion block technique with a posterior anatomic approach: the needle was introduced dorsally and forwarded through the vertebrae till the anterior

(translated by Chiara Barbaglia)

S. Savastano (✉) · E. Baldi
Division of Cardiology, Arrhythmology and Electrophysiology Unit,
Fondazione IRCCS Policlinico San Matteo, Pavia, Italy
e-mail: S.Savastano@smatteo.pv.it

S. Savastano (ed.), *Percutaneous Stellate Ganglion Block for Electrical Storm*,
https://doi.org/10.1007/978-3-031-81762-5_7

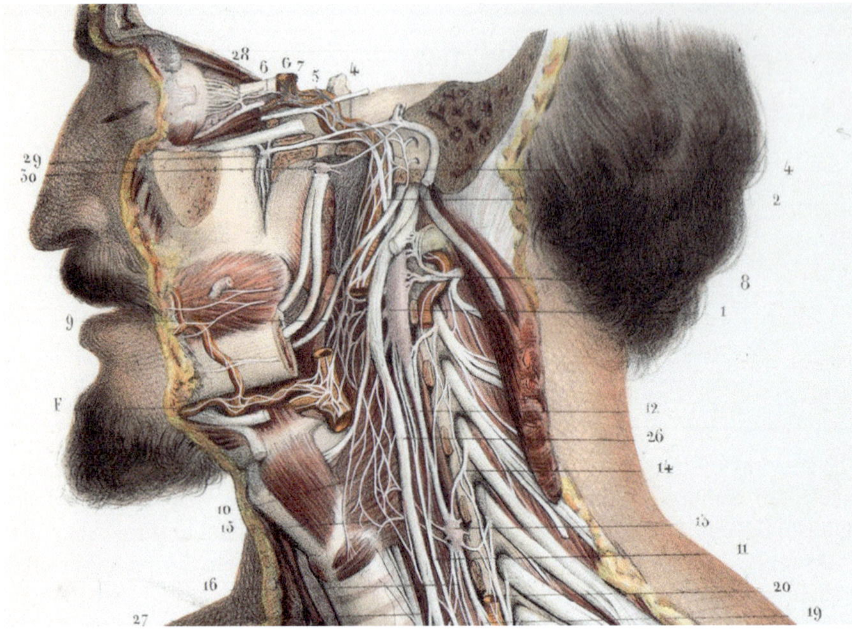

Fig. 7.1 Royal College of Physicians detail of "Nevrologie" by Jean-Baptiste Léveillé on anatomical preparation by Ludwik Hirschfeld (1816–1876). Stellate ganglion is represented at point 13. Public domain

paravertebral plane, covering a long and complex course interrupted by many anatomical structures.

The posterior approach was soon abandoned and substituted by the antero-lateral approach—developed by Leriche, Fontaine and Ochsner [4]—which was simpler and had fewer complications: the access was at the height of vertebra C7–T1, immediately over the clavicle, towards the spinal column (Fig. 7.2).

Albeit simpler and more direct than the posterior one, as it did not request side-lying for patients, the anterior supraclavicular approach frequently developed pneumothorax, as the course of the needle passed very close the pulmonary dome; damages to the vertebral artery occurred, and, after branching off the subclavian artery, its course is not protected by the transverse processes of the cervical vertebrae. In 1944, Murphey [4] perfected the technique with a new antero-lateral approach from the cricoid cartilage, but though risk-free for the lung—as inserted at a safe distance (Fig. 7.3)—the needle's course was long enough to intersect more than one vascular structure. Substituted by the anterior paratracheal approach subject of this chapter, Murphy's technique was later re-introduced and performed with the support of imaging, significantly reducing the risk of complications.

The anterior paratracheal approach was first described by Moore in 1954 [2, 6] and required the patient to lie supine with the head in hyperextension without any support; the hyperextension of the head allowed the oesophagus to collapse but

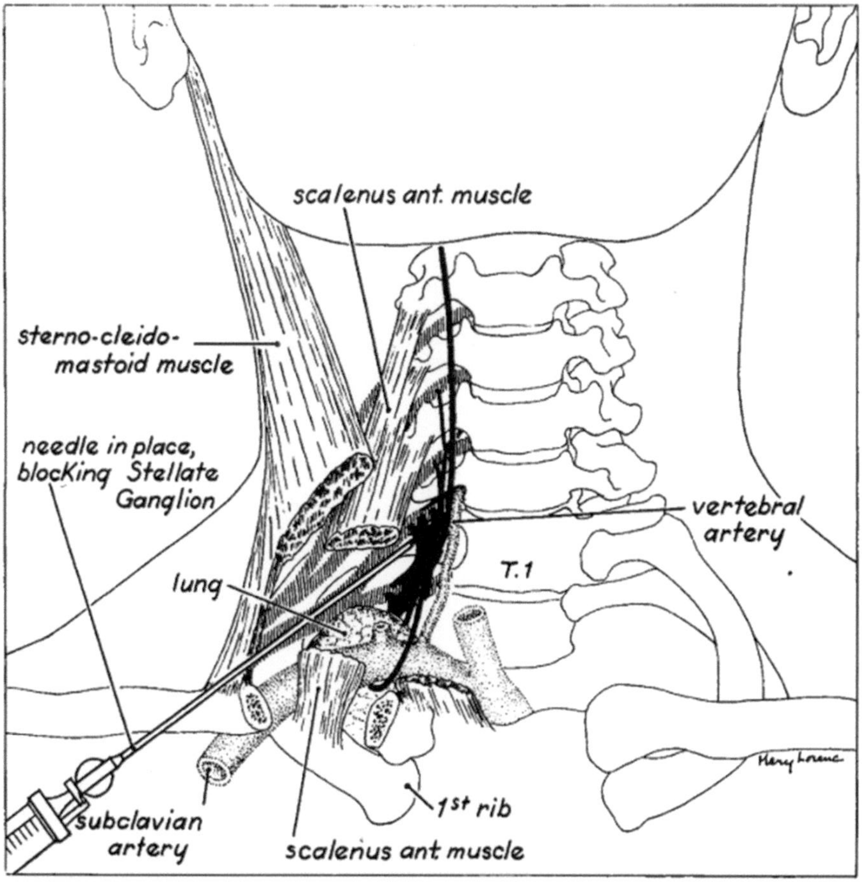

Fig. 7.2 Orkin et al. [5]—anterior supraclavicular approach

deprived the vertebral artery of the protection of the transverse processes of the cervical vertebrae: as shown in Fig. 7.4, the transverse processes of the cervical vertebrae diverge with the hyperextension and converge with the flexion of the neck. For this, in these last years, the patient's head has been kept in a neutral, non-hyperextended position, considering the risks for the vertebral artery much higher than those for the oesophagus.

Starting from the base of the neck, going two fingers up and then two fingers leftward, we are at the level of the cricoid cartilage and in the furrow bounded laterally by the sternal head of the sternocleidomastoid muscle and medially by the larynx and trachea. Deepening the fingers in the furrow, we touch the tubercle of Chassaignac (Figs. 7.5 and 7.6), the anterior tubercle of the transverse process of the sixth cervical vertebra.

As shown in Fig. 7.5, a peculiarity of this approach is the displacement of the vascular structures that are moved aside from the site of injection, so reducing and even

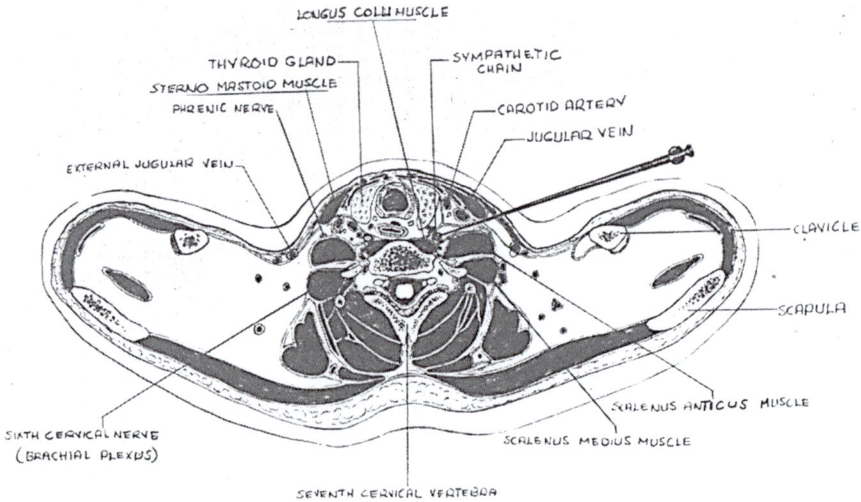

Fig. 7.3 From Murphy et al. [4]

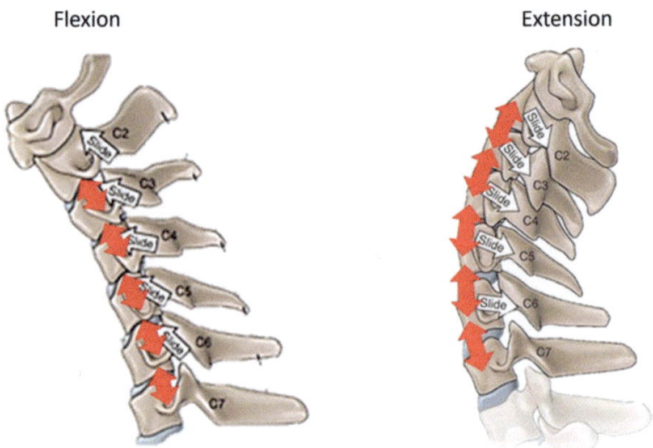

Fig. 7.4 Representation of the flexion and extension of the neck and the corresponding converging and diverging of the transversal processes

nullifying the risk of vascular complications. Once identified the Chassaignac tubercle and shifted the sternal head of the sternocleidomastoid muscle from the median line, the needle must be inserted—perpendicularly to the horizontal plane where the patient lies—till it reaches the bone. After reaching the bone, the needle must be retracted for a few millimetres to avoid injecting the periosteum, and an aspiration test must be performed to avoid intravascular injection; at this point, the anaesthetic can be administered. As shown in Fig. 7.4, although the stellate ganglion lies a bit more caudally with respect to the site of injection, the anaesthetic reaches the nerve fibres thanks to its own volume and, possibly, to the elevation of the head of the patient.

Displacing the vascular structures and touching the tubercle with the fingertips, the operator can perform the procedure in full safety, as the course of the needle in the subcutaneous tissue consists in the few millimetres between the operator's

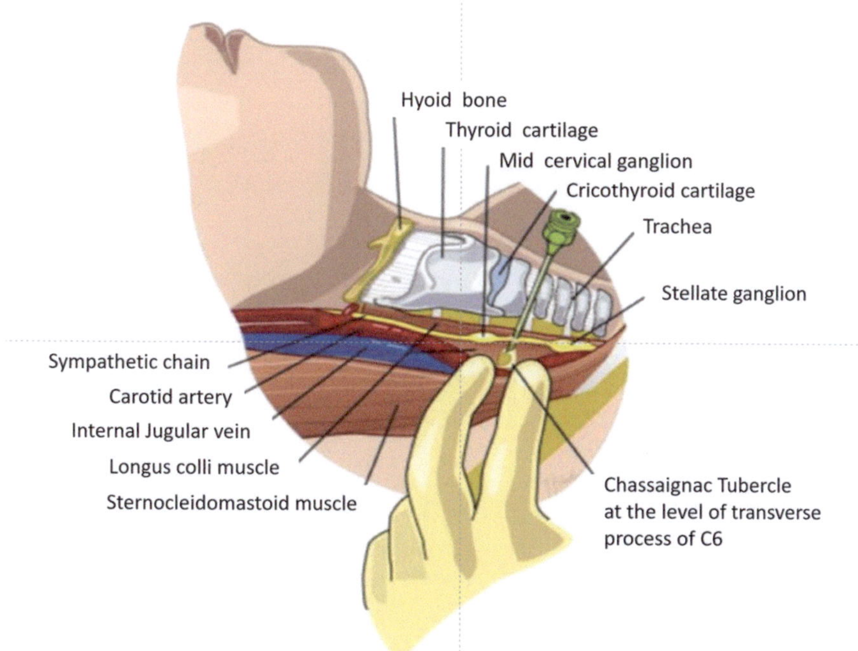

Fig. 7.5 Representation of the tubercle of Chassaignac and of its anatomical connection with the stellate ganglion

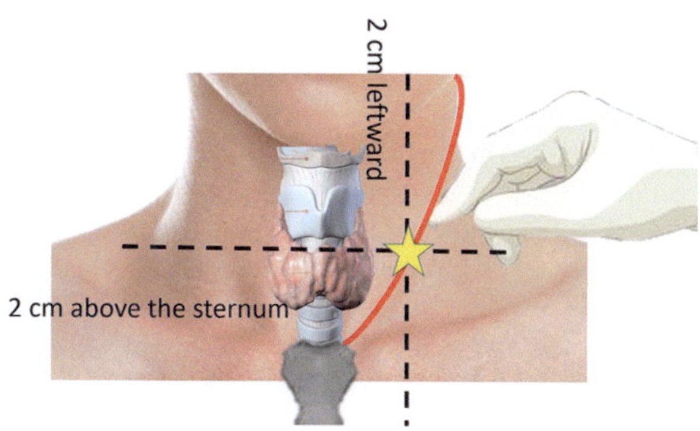

Fig. 7.6 Site of injection for the anterior anatomical approach

fingers and the target bone (Fig. 7.7). In case the bone can't be reached immediately, we recommend not inserting the needle for more than 1–1.5 cm but removing it and trying a second injection.

As the ganglion lies more caudally with respect to vertebra C6, a study of 1991 Matsumoto [7] assumed that an injection closer to the base of the neck, at the height of C7, would be more effective, but his theory was strongly debated: in absence of the anatomical landmarks necessary to locate C7, the procedure must be performed with the support of fluoroscopy. In 2005, Vallejo et al. [8] proposed a new method

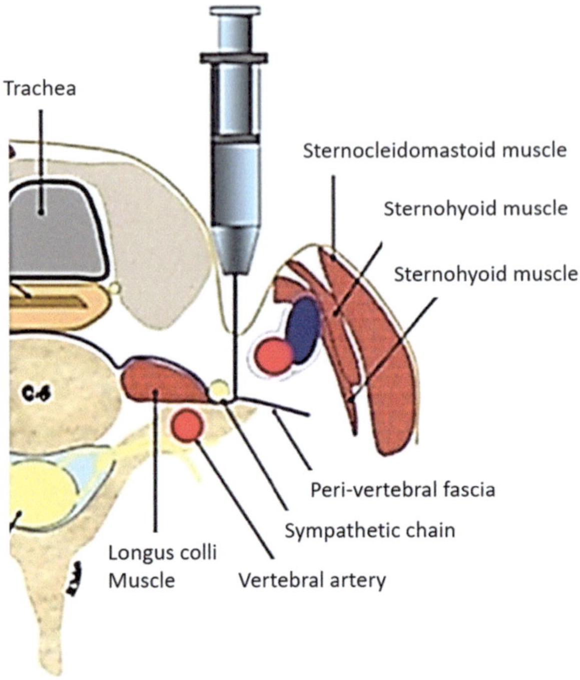

Fig. 7.7 Representation of a cross-section at the height of the tubercle of Chassaignac showing the displacement of the vascular bundle of the neck and the safe course created for the needle

that—supported by fluoroscopy—would also imply the block of T2 and T3, but further evidences, both on living [9] patient and on corpse [10], showed that the thoracic fibres can't be reached by the anaesthetic injected from the front. An interesting study by Hogan et al. [11] described—with the support of MRI—the spread of the anaesthetic and the sites of its effect after injection by anterior paratracheal approach (Fig. 7.8).

As described in Fig. 7.8, determinant to the action of the anaesthetic is the intersection of the peri-vertebral fascia (Fig. 7.7): when the peri-vertebral fascia is not crossed by the needle and the injection occurs above the fascia itself, the spreading develops in an anterior, posterior/contralateral and lateral direction (Fig. A (*I*)). Should the needle cross the peri-vertebral fascia, the anaesthetic will spread as shown in (*II*) and will be injected in the longus colli muscle [11] or in the pre-vertebral space between the peri-vertebral fascia and the vertebral bodies.

The contralateral diffusion *(I)* is more frequent in cases of injection of big volumes of anaesthetic or of repeated block procedures [12] and is a useful approach for bilateral stellate ganglion blocks; besides, it could also account for the absence of anisocoria for the occurrence of bilateral myosis.

In a study on corpse of 2000 [13], Honma et al. demonstrated how in the anterior paratracheal approach the injection occurs in the pre-vertebral space in 86% cases; in these cases, spreading through the peri-vertebral fascia, the anaesthetic reaches the ganglion in 87% cases. From a practical point of view, for the easier disconnection of structures, an injection above the peri-vertebral fascia should find a lower resistance than an intramuscular injection; for this, we suggest retracting the needle some millimetres more in case some resistance is perceived.

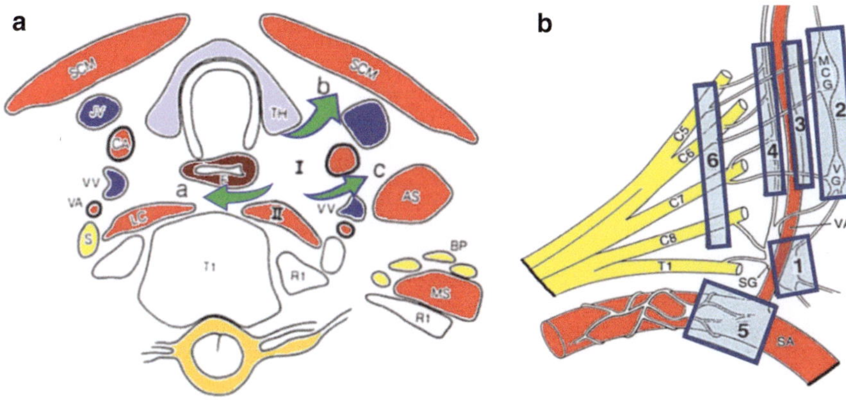

Fig. 7.8 Adaptation from Hogan et al. [11] showing the spread and the sites of action of the anaesthetic in the anterior paratracheal approach. Left—(fig **a**) green arrows indicate two possible ways of diffusion of the spread; (I) anterior (a), posterior/contralateral, (b) and a lateral (c); (II) intramuscular spread along the long muscle of the neck. Right—(fig **b**) the six sites of action of the anaesthetic: 1, stellate ganglion; 2, middle cervical (MCG) and ventral ganglion; 3, communicating nerve branches; 4, vertebral plexus; 5, subclavian plexus; 6, bronchial plexus

Either remaining in the peri-vertebral or reaching the pre-vertebral space, in the highly vascularised area of the neck, part of the anaesthetic is absorbed and circulates in the body. Among the very few studies about this topic, the one by Hardy et al. [14] measured the plasmatic concentration of bupivacaine after injection of 10 ml and 20 ml of 0.25% solution by Moore's technique. The study demonstrated that the plasmatic concentration of bupivacaine was higher after administration of 20 ml, although it was much lower than the toxic amount of 1.5 µg/ml. In the cases described by Wulf et al. [15], less than 2% patients exceeded the established toxic concentration of 2 µg/ml.

The anterior paratracheal approach, thanks to the ease of execution, the level of effectiveness and the evidences of safety, documented—though to a limited extent—even for paediatric cases, has substituted the previous techniques and has become the standard anatomical approach to percutaneous stellate ganglion block [16–18]. Its rare and non-serious complications are described in the last chapter.

References

1. Marcer N, Bergmann M, Klie A, Moor B, Djonov V. An anatomical investigation of the cervicothoracic ganglion. Clin Anat. 2012;25(4):444–51. https://doi.org/10.1002/CA.21266.
2. Walls WKJ. The anatomical approach in Stellate Ganglion Injection. 27, 1955. https://doi.org/10.1093/bja/27.12.616.
3. White JC. Angina pectoris: relief of pain by paravertebral alcohol block of the upper dorsal sympathetic rami. Arch Neurol Psychiatr. 1929;22(2):302–12. https://doi.org/10.1001/ARCHNEURPSYC.1929.02220020118007.
4. David Murphey MR, Tampa A. Stellate ganglion block: a new anterior approach. Ann Surg. 1944;120(5):759. https://doi.org/10.1097/00000658-194411000-00008.

5. Orkin LR, Papper EM, Rovenstine EA. The complications of stellate and thoracic sympathetic nerve blocks. J Thorac Surg. 1950;20(6):911–22. https://doi.org/10.1016/s0096-5588(20)31669-x.
6. Moore Daniel C. Stellate Ganglion Block: Techniques, Indications, Uses. Springfield, Ill., Thomas: N.p., 1954. Print.
7. Matsumoto S. Thermographic assessments of the sympathetic blockade by stellate ganglion block (1) comparison between C7-SGB and C6-SGB in 40 patients. Masui. 1991;40(4):562–9.
8. Vallejo R, Plancarte R, Benyamin RM, Santiago-Palma J. Anterior cervical approach for stellate ganglion and T2 to T3 sympathetic blocks: a novel technique. Pain Pract. 2005;5(3):244–8. https://doi.org/10.1111/J.1533-2500.2005.05309.X.
9. Hardy PAJ, Wells JCD. Extent of sympathetic blockade after stellate ganglion block with bupivacaine. Pain. 1989;36(2):193–6. https://doi.org/10.1016/0304-3959(89)90023-7.
10. Guntamukkala M, Hardy PAJ. Spread of injectate after stellate ganglion block in man: an anatomical study. Br J Anaesth. 1991;66(6):643–4. https://doi.org/10.1093/bja/66.6.643.
11. Hogan QH, Erickson SJ, Haddox JD, Abram SE. The spread of solutions during stellate ganglion block. Reg Anesth. 1992;17(2):78–83. PMID: 1581263.
12. Wallace MS, Milholland AV. Contralateral spread of local anesthetic with Stellate Ganglion block. Reg Anesth. 1993;18(1):55–9. https://doi.org/10.1136/rapm-00115550-199318010-00012.
13. Honma M, Murakami G, Sato TJ, Namiki A. Spread of injectate during C6 stellate ganglion block and fascial arrangement in the prevertebral region: an experimental study using donated cadavers. Reg Anesth Pain Med. 2000;25(6):573–83. https://doi.org/10.1053/RAPM.2000.8935.
14. Hardy PAJ, Williams NE. Plasma concentrations of bupivacaine after stellate ganglion block using two volumes of 0.25% bupivacaine plain solution. Br J Anaesth. 1990;65(2):243–4. https://doi.org/10.1093/bja/65.2.243.
15. Wulf H, Maier C, Schele HA, Wabbel W. Plasma concentration of bupivacaine after stellate ganglion blockade. Anesth Analg. 1991;72(4):546–8. https://doi.org/10.1213/00000539-199104000-00022.
16. Parris WCV, Reddy BC, White HW, McGrath DM. Stellate ganglion blocks in pediatric patients. Anesth Analg. 1991;72(4):552–6. https://doi.org/10.1213/00000539-199104000-00024.
17. Mesa A, Kaplan RF. Dysrhythmias controlled with stellate ganglion block in a child with diabetes and a variant of long QT syndrome. Reg Anesth. 1993;18(1):60–2.
18. Franklin AD, Llobet JR, Sobey CM, Daniels JM, Kannankeril PJ. Stellate ganglion catheter effective for treatment of ventricular tachycardia storm in a pediatric patient on extracorporeal membrane oxygenation: a case report. A&A Pract. 2019;13(7):245–9. https://doi.org/10.1213/XAA.0000000000001036.

8 Lateral Ultrasound-Guided Approach

Vito Sgromo, Enrico Contri, and Alessandra Palo

Ultrasound imaging, due to its rapidity, portability, absence of radiation and relatively low cost, represents a valuable aid for performing the stellate ganglion block.

The lateral approach recommended in this manual does not interfere with the nerves and vascular structures of the neck but highlights them, helping to avoid possible complications.

Several studies show how the lateral ultrasound-guided approach increases the effectiveness of the stellate ganglion block by injecting and spreading the anaesthetic within the prevertebral fascia (Fig. 8.1).

The ultrasound-guided approach increases the safety of the procedure thanks to direct visualisation of the surrounding anatomical structures, minimising the risk of damages [1].

In their study of 2009, Gofeld et al. [2] analysed the anatomy and location of the stellate ganglion both by cadaver dissection and MRI and CT scan. The stellate ganglion is a 1–2.5-cm-long, about 1-cm-wide and about 0.5-cm-thick structure, located anteriorly to the transverse process of C7 and superiorly and anteriorly to the insertion of the first rib.

The prevertebral fascia goes from the basis of the skull to the level of T4 covering the prevertebral muscles; the cervical sympathetic chain and, likewise, the stellate ganglion are located within this fascia and superficially to the longus colli muscle.

As a result, stellate ganglion block's effectiveness is directly related to the execution of an intra-fascial anaesthetic injection but, at the same time, is limited by a possible intramuscular diffusion of the liquid. Owing to the peculiar anatomy of this

---

(translated by Chiara Barbaglia)

V. Sgromo (✉) · E. Contri · A. Palo
Fondazione IRCCS Policlinico San Matteo, Pavia, Italy

AREU Lombardia, AAT 118, Pavia, Italy
e-mail: v.sgromo@smatteo.pv.it

S. Savastano (ed.), *Percutaneous Stellate Ganglion Block for Electrical Storm*,
https://doi.org/10.1007/978-3-031-81762-5_8

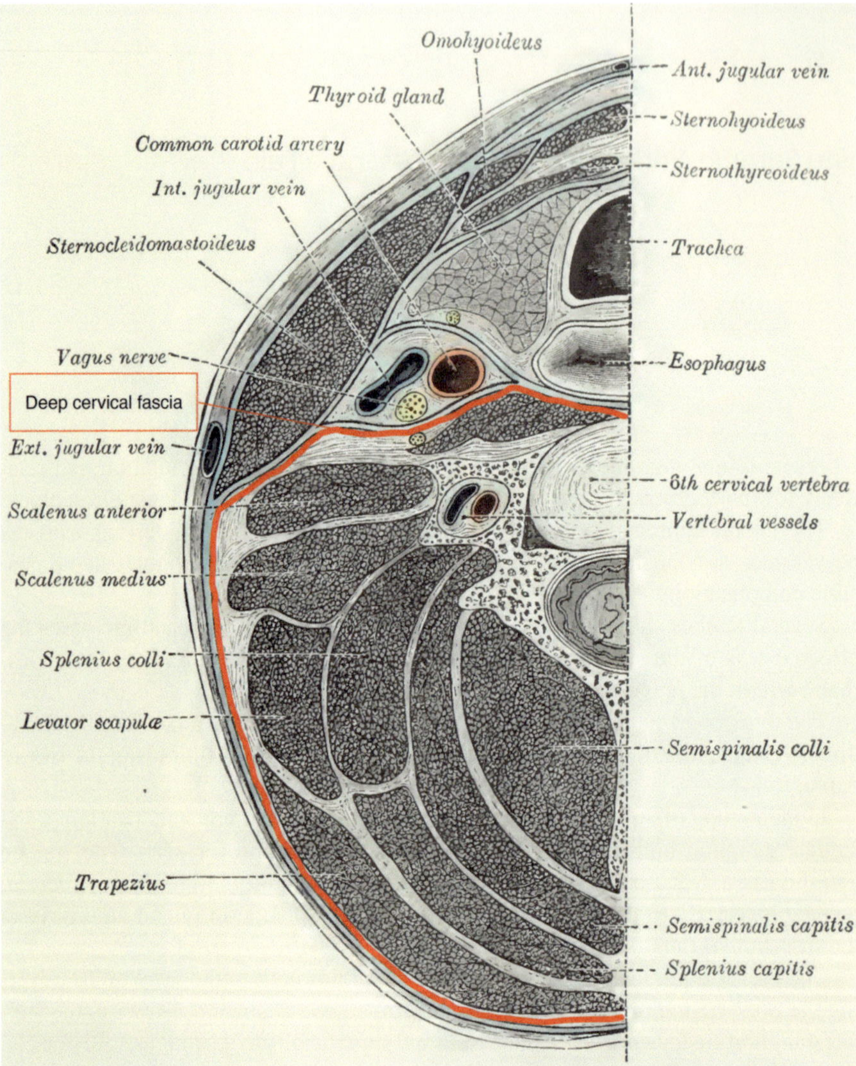

Fig. 8.1 Detail of the anatomy of the neck with the prevertebral fascia highlighted in red. (Modified from Gray H. *Anatomy of the human body*. Lea & Febiger. 1918; 389)

area and to an incorrect visualisation of the structures, a puncture of the longus colli might result in an intramuscular diffusion of the drug rather than in an infusion to the ganglion.

By the lateral ultrasound-guided approach, operators can insert the needle in an extra-muscular but still intra-fascial area, crossing and overcoming the anterior scalene muscle.

Studies on cadavers have shown that only the administration of the anaesthetic in the sub-fascial space allows an adequate diffusion of the anaesthetic to the stellate ganglion.

Technique

The patient lies supine, and his neck is rotated in opposite direction to the site of injection [3] (Fig. 8.2).

Since we seek to visualise superficial structures located a few centimetres from the skin, we recommend using a high-frequency (8–12 MHz) linear probe [4].

After skin and probe disinfection, we place the transducer obliquely between C6 and C7. The image we need to obtain should be as close as possible to our ideal and clearly display: the sternocleidomastoid muscle in the proximal part of the probe, the anterior scalene muscle in the needle entry side, the internal jugular vein and the carotid artery in front of the site of injection, the longus colli (often not visible at echo) and the vertebral plane in the lower part of the screen (Fig. 8.3).

These structures delimit an area where we can inject—safely and with a high success rate—the local anaesthetic in the direction of the longus colli above which the cervical sympathetic chain and the stellate ganglion lie.

Depending on the ultrasound slice, we can also visualise the thyroid gland and vertebral vessels (Fig. 8.4).

The use of colour Doppler in a preliminary scan can help detecting any abnormal vessels or any important anatomical variant along the needle course.

The needle, preferably between 5 and 8 cm long, should have a high degree of reflectivity in order to be clearly visible throughout its course.

Then, keeping the in-plane visualisation (long axis), we insert the needle posteriorly, and, after passing through the anterior scalene muscle, we directed it towards the longus colli without penetrating it.

By crossing the anterior scalene muscle, we can pass the prevertebral fascia injecting the anaesthetic close to the longus colli, above which the cervical sympathetic chain and the stellate ganglion are located (Fig. 8.5).

At this point, we can inject the local anaesthetic and, if we are in the correct area (intra-fascial but outside the longus colli), a volume of 10 ml will be enough to reach and block the stellate ganglion (Fig. 8.6).

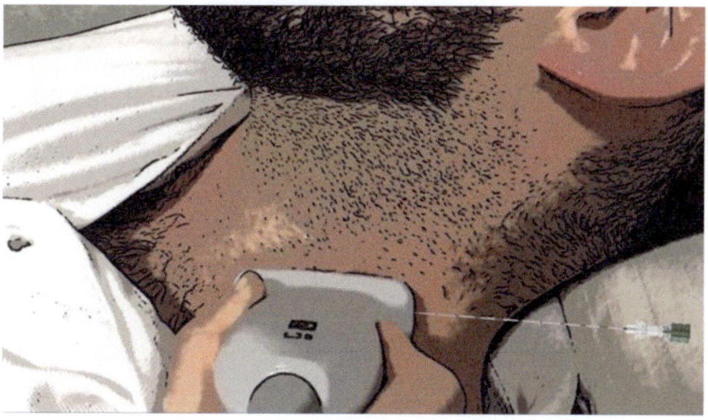

Fig. 8.2 Lateral ultrasound approach. The position of the needle is highlighted

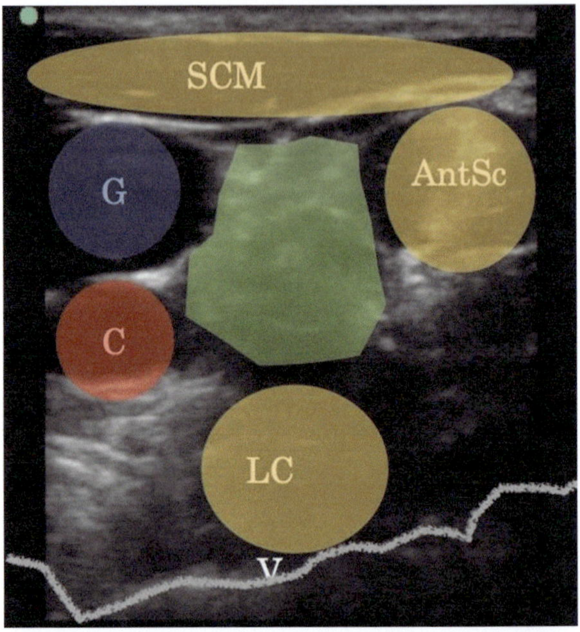

Fig. 8.3 In yellow, the sternocleidomastoid (SCM), anterior scalene (AntSc) and longus colli (LC) muscles. In blue, the jugular vein (G). In red, the carotid artery (C). In white, the vertebral plane (V). In green, the puncture site

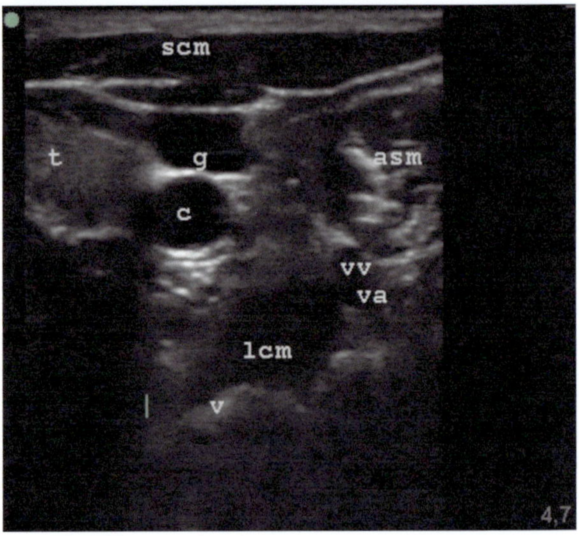

Fig. 8.4 Ultrasound image at the level of C6–C7. *scm* sternocleidomastoid, *asm* anterior scalene muscle, *lcm* longus colli muscle, *t* thyroid, *g* jugular, *c* carotid, *vv* vertebral vein, *va* vertebral artery, *v* vertebral plane

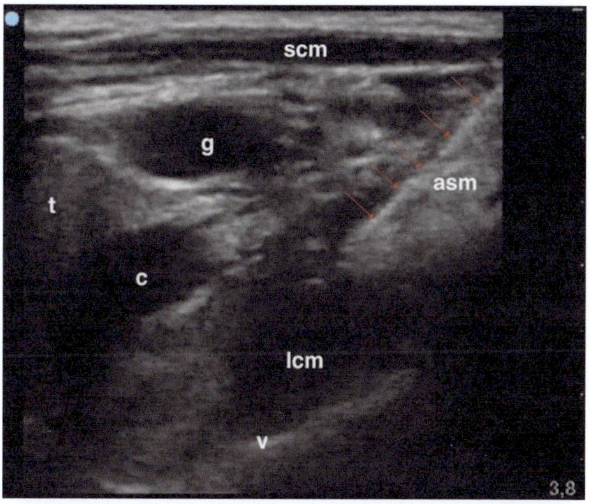

Fig. 8.5 Puncture and crossing of the anterior scalene muscle. Needle indicated by red arrows

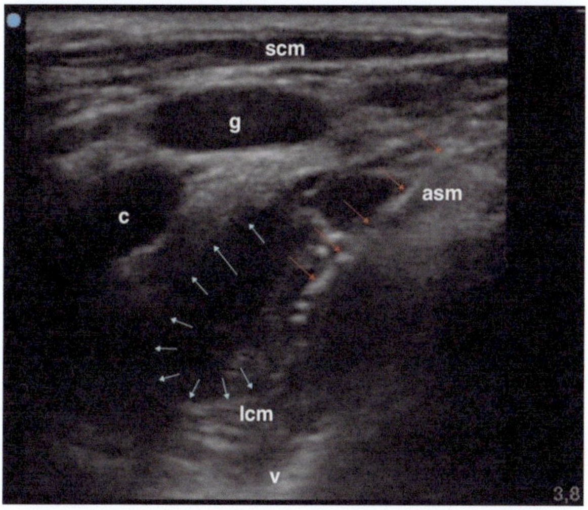

Fig. 8.6 Injection of local anaesthetic and its diffusion. The red arrows indicate the needle, and the blue arrows mark the area of anaesthetic diffusion

Complications

It has been shown how ultrasound could prevent the possible complications of stellate ganglion block by identifying the structures most at risk of damage (vertebral vessels, thyroid vessels and gland, oesophagus and nerve roots). It is thus possible to reduce the risk of retropharyngeal haematomas caused by the puncture of the thyroid or vertebral artery; the latter enters the foramen of the transverse process above C6 in about 10% of cases and is therefore more vulnerable [5].

The oesophagus, which runs more laterally rather than posteriorly to the cricoid and trachea in about 50% of cases, can also be identified by ultrasound, preventing its accidental puncture and the consequent risk of mediastinal infection and/or emphysema.

The use of ultrasounds may also prevent the block of the recurrent laryngeal nerve as the lateral ultrasound-guided approach implies that the puncture is far enough from the nerve.

Here you can access the educational video on Percutaneous Left Stellate Ganglion Block for Electrical Storm.

References

1. Ghai A, Kaushik T, Kundu ZS, Wadhera S, Wadhera R. Evaluation of new approach to ultrasound guided stellate ganglion block. Saudi J Anaesth. 2016;10(2):161–7.
2. Gofeld M, Bhatia A, Abbas S, Ganapathy S, Johnson M. Development and validation of a new technique for ultrasound-guided stellate ganglion block. Reg Anesth Pain Med. 2009;34(5):475–9.
3. Chang KV, Wu WT, Özçakar L. Ultrasound-guided interventions of the cervical spine and nerves. Phys Med Rehabil Clin N Am. 2018;29(1):93–103.
4. Serna-Gutiérrez J. Bloqueo ganglio estrellado guiado por ultrasonografia. Rev Colomb Anesthesiol. 2015;43:278–82.
5. Narouze S, Vydyanathan A, Patel N. Ultrasound-guided stellate ganglion block successfully prevented esophageal puncture. Pain Physician. 2007;10(6):747–52.

Part IV

Additional Considerations

Pharmacology of Local Anaesthetics

9

Alessia Currao and Simone Savastano

Local anaesthesia is the condition that occurs when sensory afference from a specific region of the body to the Central Nervous System (CNS) is effectively blocked.

Local anaesthetics represent a heterogeneous class of drugs whose main purpose is to bring about the blockage of nerve impulse conduction by inducing loss of sensation (anaesthesia) in a specific body district, allowing the physician to intervene on the patient. Local anaesthetic drugs, unlike general anaesthetics, do not lead to a loss of consciousness, but their action remains regionally limited to the site of delivery [1, 2].

Mechanism of Action of Local Anaesthetics

The specific receptor theory, currently the most widely accepted, posits that local anaesthetics act by binding to specific sites on sodium channels expressed on the neuronal membrane. The neuronal membrane is the site where local anaesthetics exert their pharmacological actions. The action of local anaesthetics is direct, not mediated by changes in membrane properties. In the sodium channel, there is a specific binding site for local anaesthetics on its outer surface or on the inner axoplasmic surface. Once the local anaesthetic has gained access to this site, sodium ion permeability is either decreased or eliminated, resulting in the interruption of nerve conduction.

A. Currao (✉)
Division of Cardiology, Fondazione IRCCS Policlinico San Matteo, Pavia, Italy

Department of Internal Medicine and Medical Therapy, University of Pavia, Pavia, Italy
e-mail: a.currao@smatteo.pv.it

S. Savastano
Division of Cardiology, Arrhythmology and Electrophysiology Unit, Fondazione IRCCS Policlinico San Matteo, Pavia, Italy

S. Savastano (ed.), *Percutaneous Stellate Ganglion Block for Electrical Storm*,
https://doi.org/10.1007/978-3-031-81762-5_9

The mechanism of action of local anaesthetic drugs, therefore, involves the blocking (transient and reversible) voltage-dependent Na^+ channels (Na_v), located on the neuronal membrane. This results in a reduction in the influx of Na^+ ions, thereby preventing the normal depolarisation of the neuronal membrane. Consequently, the generation and propagation of the electrical action potential and, therefore, the conduction of the nerve impulse are prevented (Fig. 9.1).

It has been demonstrated that many local anaesthetics exert 'use-dependent' blocking effects on Na^+ channels, i.e. the intensity of channel block increases as the frequency of action potentials increases. This results in an increase in the arousal threshold, a slowing of the impulse conduction velocity, a reduction in the amplitude of the action potential and the cessation of action potentials propagation along the nerve fibre. The *use-dependency* may be particularly important in the context of stellate ganglion block, as arrhythmic storm is known to be a condition that results in an activation of the sympathetic nervous system and thus an increased number of impulses along nerve fibres.

Local anaesthetics act by locally inhibiting the conduction of action potentials in all afferent and efferent nerve fibres of the peripheral nervous system.

Different types of nerve fibres are blocked at different times following the administration of the local anaesthetic depending on the concentration gradient of the anaesthetic within the nerve and the characteristics of the nerve fibre. In fact, the differential sensitivity of different types of nerve fibres to local anaesthetics depends on the following factors:

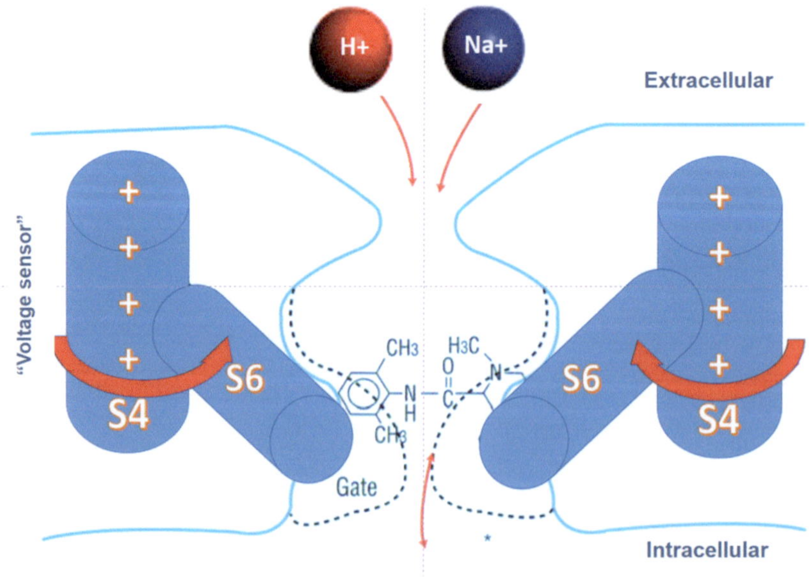

Fig. 9.1 A schematic representation of the mechanism of action of local anaesthetics. Note how the binding of the local anaesthetic to the sodium channel prevents the conformational changes normally due to the passage of sodium ions

- *Fibre diameter:* fibres with a smaller diameter are more easily blocked than fibres with a larger diameter.
- *Myelination (or lack thereof) of the fibres:* myelinated fibres are blocked more easily than unmyelinated ones, as impulse conduction is considerably faster and more efficient. Furthermore, the densities of sodium channels differ between myelinated (higher) and unmyelinated (lower) nerves.
- *Fibre discharge frequency:* nociceptive fibres discharge at a high frequency when activated. This suggests that local anaesthetics may selectively block nociceptive sensation.
- *Anatomical location of the fibres:* fibres located peripherally are blocked more rapidly than those located within the core of a nerve bundle, as they are exposed earlier to high concentrations of anaesthetic.

The duration of action of local anaesthetics is proportional to the time they remain in contact with the nerve. The lowest dose deemed effective in inducing the desired effect (the blockade) is therefore recommended [1–3].

Chemical and Physical Properties Underlying the Pharmacological Effects of Local Anaesthetics

Local anaesthetics are characterised by common structural chemical features. All molecules are characterised by three chemical groups:

- An *unsaturated aromatic structure* (benzoic or para-aminobenzoic acid), which imparts fat solubility to the molecule.
- An *intermediate chain* consisting of an ester ($-COO^-$) or amide (-CONH) bond.
- A *tertiary* (or, rarely, *secondary*) *amine derivative* of ethyl alcohol or acetic acid, which imparts the molecule with the properties of weak base and hydrophilicity.

Depending on the type of intermediate chain, local anaesthetics are then subdivided into:

- *Esters*, which are characterised by a short duration of action, as esters bonds are quickly hydrolysed by plasma cholinesterases; these substances are also unstable in solution.
- *Amides*, which undergo slow hepatic metabolism, which explaining their prolonged action and the appearance of active metabolites. Since the amide bond is much more stable than the ester bond, the solution is resistant to heat and pH changes. Lidocaine is the prototypical local anaesthetic of the amide group.

With regard to therapeutic use, local anaesthetics are usually supplied as salts (typically as chlorides, Cl^-) for reasons of solubility and stability.

The local anaesthetic in the human body is present in two forms: a basic, fat-soluble undissociated form and a dissociated (cationic) water-soluble form. Both forms contribute to the action of local anaesthetics since the fat-soluble, indissociated form is the only one that crosses the membrane and is therefore responsible for the penetration of the local anaesthetic into nerve sheaths and axonal membranes. The cationic form plays the primary role as it binds reversibly to the receptors in the sodium channel and reducing their conductance, thus exerting the actual action of the drug.

In the body, the relative proportions of these two forms are present depending on the respective pK and pH of the body fluids (as described by the *Henderson–Hasselbalch equation*). Since the pKa of local anaesthetics is between 8 and 9, the most consistent fraction in body fluids at physiological pH is the ionised (cationic) form. It is considered the most active form at the receptor site as it is not easily metabolised at the level of blocked ion channels; the non-ionised fraction is, moreover, crucial for rapid passage across biological membranes. Hence, their activity is strongly influenced by pH.

Liposolubility, protein binding and pKa therefore represent key pharmacological factors for each local anaesthetic. Specifically:

- *Liposolubility* determines the potency of local anaesthetics: anaesthetics with higher liposolubility are generally also the most potent. This is related to their ability to easily cross the phospholipid bilayer of cell membranes.
- *Protein binding* has a significant effect on the duration of blockade. A large percentage of protein-bound local anaesthetics exhibit a high binding affinity for receptor proteins. The local anaesthetics with the highest potency also tend to have the longest duration of action.
  Longer-acting local anaesthetics (bupivacaine, ropivacaine, etc.) are more tightly bound to the nerve membrane (exhibiting higher protein binding) than shorter-acting drugs (lidocaine), and are therefore released more slowly from sodium channel receptor sites.
- The *pKa*, defined as the pH at which 50% of the drug is present in the ionised form and 50% in the non-ionised form, is crucial in determining the *onset of action*. Anaesthetics with a pKa close to physiological pH will have a faster onset because they are present in solution—predominantly—in the non-ionised (base) portion. As the pK increases, the ionised portion will prevail in solution, which is responsible for a slower *onset*.

The basic, fat-soluble form is responsible for interaction with the components of the cellular lipid bilayer and conditions perinervous diffusion, while the ionised, hydrophilic form governs the pharmacological effect following cellular entry of the local anaesthetic [2–5]. (Table 9.1).

Table 9.1 Pharmacological properties of the main local anaesthetic agents [1, 2, 6–17]

Local anaesthetic	Onset time of action	Duration of action	Half-life ($t_{½}$)	Safe and effective dose in PSGB	Recommended maximum dose[a]
Lidocaine	Rapid	Medium	~2 h	**Bolus**: 200 mg in 10 ml; (conc. 2% by volume 8–12 ml) **Infusion**: Lidocaine 1.67 mg/min (200 mg every 2 h) Alternatively, association of: lidocaine 200 mg + bupivacaine 50 mg by volume 20 ml	6 mg/kg In the healthy adult (not pretreated with sedatives) the maximum dose, in a single administration or in several repeated administrations, is 300 mg total in less than 120 min.
Mepivacaine	Rapid	Medium	~2 h	**Bolus**: 100 mg in 10 ml; (conc. 1% by volume 10 ml)	Do not exceed a dose of 300 mg per session. The maximum dose in the healthy adult (not pretreated with sedatives), as a single administration or in several repeated administrations over a period of less than 90 min, is 7 mg/kg without ever exceeding 550 mg. The total dose over 24 h must never exceed 1000 mg.

(continued)

Table 9.1 (continued)

Local anaesthetic	Onset time of action	Duration of action	Half-life ($t_{½}$)	Safe and effective dose in PSGB	Recommended maximum dose[a]
Bupivacaine	Medium	Long	~3.5 h	**Bolus**: 50 mg in 10 ml; (conc. 0.5% by volume 10 ml)	– The indication for use in 'stellate ganglion blockade' is approved by the Italian Medicines Agency (AIFA) with the following indications for guidance: conc. 0.25%; dosage 10–20 ml/25–50 mg. – It is usually used in minimum dosages, varying according to indication, from 2–3 mg to 100–150 mg. – The maximum dosage (for adult, per single administration) should not exceed 150 mg; more generally, the safe dose that should not be exceeded is 2 mg/kg per single administration. In prolonged analgesic therapy, doses ranging from 0.25 to 1 mg/kg body weight are usually used; administration may be repeated two to three times over 24 h.
Ropivacaine	Slow	Long	~4.2 h	Conc. 0.5–0.75% in 10 ml; **Bolus**: lidocaine 200 mg + ropivacaine 50 mg **Infusion**: Ropivacaine 0.2 mg/min (12 mg/h)	3 mg/kg (max. 225–300 mg)

Prilocaine	Rapid	Medium	~2 h	Possible indication of use in the PSGB Evidence of use in the literature, e.g. in stellate ganglion block for the treatment of pain [18, 19]	6 mg/kg in adults (max. 400 mg)

[a]The dose to be administered should also be based on the physician's experience and knowledge of the patient's clinical condition. Dosage should be determined on an individual basis. The minimum doses and concentrations necessary to achieve an effective block should always be employed. The doses provided in the table are those deemed necessary to produce an adequate block and should be considered as a guide for use in adults (avg weight ~70 kg). However, individual variations in the timing and duration may occur. The spread of anaesthesia can be difficult to predict, though it is influenced by the volume of the drug administered. Administration of local anaesthetics should be discontinued immediately if signs of acute systemic toxicity appear. Injections into inflamed or infected areas should be avoided. The 'Average dose in PSGB' column indicates the typical dose ranges employed in the PSGB procedure [9–17] (www.aifa.gov.it: https://farmaci.agenziafarmaco.gov.it/bancadatifarmaci/)

Clinical Characteristics of Local Anaesthetics and Possible Associations

Local anaesthetics are commonly used for minor operations, frequently in combination with vasoconstrictors such as epinephrine. In addition to the anaesthetic effect, or more generally the blocking of nerve conduction, they also have other potentially interesting clinical effects.

For example, local anaesthetics also have antimicrobial effects, suggesting their use in prophylaxis and—in the case of bacterial resistance—in the treatment of post-procedural infection, thus allowing a wider clinical application. In addition *methylparaben*, a preservative agent commonly contained in multipurpose lidocaine vials, which has a known antibacterial activity, has been shown to enhance the antimicrobial effect of lidocaine in vitro. It is therefore believed that tissue infiltration with local anaesthetics may explain the low wound complication rate associated with minor surgery [6–8]. Lidocaine and bupivacaine also demonstrate a significant dose-dependent anti-inflammatory effect through the modulation of polymorphonuclear granulocytes (PMNGs) inhibiting the release of inflammatory mediators, such as leukotriene B4 (LTB-4) and interleukin-1 (IL-1). These findings may, therefore, explain the notably low incidence of infectious complications associated with PSGB, even in the context of prolonged infusions.

In clinical practice local anaesthetics are frequently co-administered with a vasoconstrictor, typically epinephrine, to reduce local blood flow in order to prolong the anaesthetic's residence at the target site (and consequently the anaesthetic effect) and to modulate the rate of drug metabolism in parallel with its rate of absorption into the systemic circulation, thus minimizing systemic toxicity. It follows that longer-acting anaesthetics, such as bupivacaine and ropivacaine, are less reliant on the simultaneous administration of vasoconstrictors.

In the specific case of the PSGB procedure, on the other hand, the combination of a local anaesthetic with a vasoconstrictor is not routinely practiced, as there is -to date- no scientific rationale to support a potential benefit for the patient. On the contrary, firstly, the induced local vasoconstriction could lead to a localised necrosis and tissue ischaemia, thus increasing the risk of local complications. Secondly, in the - albeit rare - case of intravascular injection or tissue absorption (remember that epinephrine can be, also, administered intramuscularly in certain clinical situations) there is a risk of exacerbating the patient's arrhythmic condition, which was originally being addressed by PSGB.

In addition to vasoconstrictors, local anaesthetics are commonly co-administered with other adjuvant agents, such as sodium bicarbonate ($NaHCO_3$) or steroidal anti-inflammatory (corticosteroids or cortisone) drugs, in order to facilitate a rapid onset of action and enhance both potency and duration of effect. Specifically *sodium bicarbonate*, through the carbonation reaction, promotes the alkalinisation of the solution, resulting in a higher proportion of the anaesthetic in its neutral (non-ionised) form, which is more capable of crossing phospholipid membranes. The optimal amount of bicarbonate to be added depends on the pKa of the anaesthetic (e.g. lidocaine pKa 7.9: 1 ml of 8.4% bicarbonate per 10 ml of solution; bupivacaine pKa 8.1: 0.1 ml of 8.4% bicarbonate per 10 ml of solution).

Corticosteroids, on the other hand, in cases of use in combination with local anaesthetics for the management of localised pain syndromes, play a more significant role as co-adjuvants, by inhibiting the inflammatory process, thereby contributing to the alleviation of pain symptoms [18]. In the specific case of PSGB, *Reinertsen* et al. [9] reported the effective use of variable combinations of bupivacaine, lidocaine and ropivacaine with dexamethasone. In addition, we also report the results of a prospective, randomised, double-blind trial aimed at evaluating the onset and duration of axillary brachial plexus blockade, in which the conjunction of dexamethasone with lidocaine was shown to prolong the duration of both sensory and motor blockade [20]. However, given the paucity of reports in literature and the absence of further robust evidence supporting the aforementioned potential associations in the specific context of PSGB for antiarrhythmic purposes, the routine clinical use of adjuvant agents in this setting cannot be recommended.

Safe and Effective Mode of Administration in PSGB [9–17]

Based on the existing literature and our own experience, we propose the following administration scheme for both bolus and infusion:

- **Bolus**
  - Single-shot injection of the anaesthetic (administered over, approximately, 1 min)
  - *Recommended dosage*: lidocaine 200 mg ± bupivacaine 50 mg or ropivacaine 50 mg.
- **Infusion**
  - Continuous injection via permanent catheter (epidural) and infusion pump connection.
  - *Recommended dosage*: lidocaine 1.67 mg/min (200 mg every 2 h). Based on our experience, we recommend preparing a solution such that 100 mg corresponds to 20 ml, thereby setting an infusion rate of 20 ml/h. Alternatively, ropivacaine 0.2 mg/min (12 mg/h).

Local Anaesthetics: Undesirable Effects and Systemic Toxicity

The undesirable effects of local anaesthetics result from their passage into the systemic circulation. Many local anaesthetics, especially short-acting ones, are readily absorbed into the bloodstream from the injection site.

Toxic systemic reactions primarily affect the central nervous system and the cardiovascular system. These reactions are caused by elevated blood concentrations of the local anaesthetic agent, which may result from an accidental intravascular injection, overdose, or exceptionally rapid absorption from a highly vascularized area. CNS reactions are consistent across all amide-type local anaesthetics, whereas cardiac reactions are more drug-dependent, both quantitatively and qualitatively.

Important effects are observed on the central nervous system, autonomic ganglia and the neuromuscular junction. The effects on the central nervous system are primarily excitatory and encompass symptoms such as agitation, tremor, progressing to convulsions and severe respiratory depression. Central nervous system toxicity typically manifests gradually, with symptoms and signs of increasing severity.

In the cardiovascular system, conversely, local anaesthetics can induce myocardial depression, characterized by a decrease in electrical excitability, conduction velocity and myocardial contractil force, as well as vasodilation, leading to hypotension. Cardiovascular toxicity is indicative of a more severe condition. Hypotension, bradycardia, arrhythmias, and even cardiac arrest may occur due to elevated systemic concentrations of local anaesthetics. Cardiovascular toxic effects are generally preceded by signs of central nervous system toxicity, unless the patient has been heavily sedated with benzodiazepines or barbiturates, or pretreated with general anaesthetics.

Hypersensitivity reactions, such as allergic dermatitis, may also occur. *Practical examples:* Lidocaine and bupivacaine, which are widely used local anaesthetics to provide a regional anaesthesia following local administration. When used topically, through local infiltration or via regional nerve block, they block the transduction and transmission of primary afferent signals. Both of these drugs exhibit cardiovascular toxic effects (e.g., arrhythmias, cardiac depression, etc.) and neurological toxic effects (e.g., convulsions), which may occur even at doses close to therapeutic levels. Furthermore, since these drugs undergo hepatic metabolism, they should be administered with particular caution in patients with liver disease or dysfunction, as prolonged drug half-life increases the risk of toxicity.

The use of levobupivacaine (the levogyric isomer of racemic bupivacaine), in contrast to bupivacaine itself would be preferable due to its favorable safety profile, particularly regarding its effects on the cardiovascular system.

However, there is a lack of comparative clinical data -to date- concerning the degree of reversibility of arrhythmias or cardiac arrest induced by these two anaesthetics.

The incidence of serious cardiac events, although low, has been further reduced over the years due to improvements in anaesthesia techniques, such as dose fractionation, use of dose-testing, careful aspiration before and during administration to avoid intravascular injection etc.) [21–33] (Table 9.2).

The prevalence of the (potential) toxicity of a local anaesthetic drug is a critical aspect in its proper consideration for clinical use. When performing prolonged peripheral nerve blocks, whether through continuous infusion or anaesthetic injections, the risk of achieving toxic concentrations and inducing local neural injury must be carefully assessed. In order to prevent intravascular administration, it is essential to aspirate repeatedly before and during the administration of the primary dose, which should be injected slowly or in progressively fractionated doses, while closely monitoring the patient's vital signs and, if possible, maintaining verbal contact. An accidental intravascular injection may be identified by a temporary increase in heart rate.

Table 9.2 Commonly used local anaesthetics: main undesirable effects, particular notes and warnings [1, 2, 6, 7, 21–28, 34]

Local anaesthetic	Main undesirable effects	Particular notes and warnings
Lidocaine	– Bradycardia, reduced cardiac output, hypotension (due to block of the sympathetic system). – Vasodilation, to the point of circulatory collapse. But *minor* tendency to cause major CNS effects (such as agitation, anxiety, chills, tremors, convulsions and respiratory depression). Undesirable effects are generally dose-dependent and may result from high plasma levels due to overdose, rapid absorption and accidental intravascular injection or may be caused by hypersensitivity or idiosyncrasy.	– Amide-type local anaesthetic. – As approved indications for use: peripheral nerve conduction block and local infiltration. – Anaesthetic solution must be injected carefully, in small doses, about 10 sec. after aspiration. – Depending on concentration, it demonstrated bacteriostatic and/or bactericidal activity against *Escherichia coli*, *Enterobacteriaceae*, *pseudomonas*, *Staphylococcus aureus 1–3* and some methicillin- and vancomycin-resistant strains. – Tissue penetration: Good – It also exhibits an anti-inflammatory properties, useful in treating pain.
Mepivacaine	– Unlike all other local anaesthetics, it does not possess vasodilating properties, which allows it to be used without a vasoconstrictor in cases where this is contraindicated. – Risk of toxicity in infants due to slow metabolism.	– Amide-type local anaesthetic. – Pharmacological properties similar to lidocaine. – Tissue penetration: Good – All liver diseases (cirrhosis, hepatitis) lead to accumulation of mepivacaine, as the liver is the main site of metabolism. – Administration is contraindicated in cases of low plasma cholinesterase levels, myasthenia gravis and severe hepatic insufficiency.

(continued)

Table 9.2 (continued)

Local anaesthetic	Main undesirable effects	Particular notes and warnings
Bupivacaine	Side effects substantially superimposed on lidocaine but *greater* cardiotoxicity.	– Amide-type local anaesthetic. – Indicated in all types of peripheral anaesthesia. – Compared to lidocaine, it has greater antibacterial activity. – Tissue penetration: Moderate – Compared to bupivacaine, **levo-bupivacaine** (enantiomer S) is less cardiotoxic and less CNS depressant and is associated with less vasodilation and longer duration of action. However, it is less potent than racemic bupivacaine, and the onset time of neuro-muscle blockade is longer. Approved indications for use of levobupivacaine include blockade of peripheral nerve conduction (and specifically for stellate ganglion blockade) and local infiltration. – It also exhibits anti-inflammatory properties, useful in treating pain.
Ropivacaine	– To be used with caution in patients with severe hepatic impairment; administration of repeated doses must be reduced due to delayed elimination. – When used as a single dose or for short-term treatment in patients with impaired renal function, there is no need to adjust the dose. – Acidosis and decreased plasma protein concentration, frequently observed in patients with chronic renal impairment, may increase the risk of systemic toxicity. – Recommend caution with class III antiarrhythmics (e.g. amiodarone).	– It is a long-acting amide local anaesthetic, which has both anaesthetic and analgesic effects. At high doses, it produces anaesthesia; at lower doses, it induces sensory blockade with limited motor blockade. – The onset of activity and duration of local anaesthetic efficacy depend on the site of administration and the dose but are not influenced by the presence of vasoconstrictors. – Does not exert additional antibacterial activity. – Compared to bupivacaine, it has less cardiotoxicity. – It is indicated in continuous peripheral nerve block for continuous infusion or intermittent bolus injections. – It should be used with caution in patients treated with other local anaesthetics or substances structurally related to amide-type local anaesthetics, e.g. certain antiarrhythmics such as lidocaine and mexiletine, as the systemic toxic effects are additive.

Prilocaine	Rare cases of clinically significant methaemoglobinaemia have been reported in cases of overdose. *Acute systemic toxicity*, cardiovascular toxicity and CNS toxicity may also occur.	– It is an amide-type local anaesthetic. – It also exhibits an anti-arrhythmic action by acting on the Na^+ channels of the Purkinje fibres. – It has low cardiotoxicity and is relatively safe in pregnant women. – For topical use, it is used in combination with lidocaine. – Tissue penetration: Moderate

Toxicity among currently used local anaesthetics varies considerably. However, the aspect that should not be underestimated is the potential for systemic toxicity, as all injectable local anaesthetics and most topical local formulations, eventually absorbed systemically, leading to cardiotoxic undesirable effects of varying severity.

Systemic absorption of the local anaesthetic from the site of administration may be influenced by the following factors:

- Administered drug-dose
- Injection site
- Drug–tissue bonding
- Presence of vasoconstrictors
- Chemical–physical and pharmacological properties of drug

The vascularisation status of the tissues influences the permanence of the drug in the target site: hyperaemia in the affected area, often associated with inflammatory processes, can result in drug concentrations comparable to those achieved through direct intravenous injection. Substances with vasoconstrictive properties, such as epinephrine and other catecholamines, are capable of reducing the systemic absorption of local anaesthetics by decreasing blood flow in the affected region; this effect is particularly pronounced with short- to intermediate-acting anaesthetics.

In plasma, local anaesthetics bind to proteins in a manner proportional to their lipophilicity. These drugs readily cross lipid structures such as cell membranes, the blood–brain barrier and the placenta, achieving higher concentrations in tissues than in the bloodstream.

The metabolism of local anaesthetics occurs primarily in the plasma or liver, with only a small fraction being excreted unchanged in the urine [1, 2].

Mulroy et al. [29] reported the incidence of systemic local anaesthetic toxicity in approximately 7.5–20/10,000 peripheral nerve blocks and in approximately 1/10,000 peridural anaesthesias. *Auroy* et al. [30] conducted a large survey among French anaesthesiologists on the complications of regional anaesthesia and reported an incidence of local anaesthetic-induced convulsions in 0–25/10,000 peripheral nerve blocks, but, surprisingly, no cardiac arrests were reported in this study. In contrast, in a more recent study *Lee* et al., [31] analysing the American Society of Anesthesiologists (ASA) Closed Claims Database from 1980 to 2000, have reported: 'local anaesthetic toxicity is a major cause of death or brain damage in these claims'. It is clear, therefore, that an accurate estimate of the incidence of severe systemic toxicity of local anaesthetics is extremely difficult and is probably higher than reported in *peer literature*. The systemic (neurological and cardiovascular) toxicity of local anaesthetics is a function of the maximum plasma concentration (Cp max) and the time interval in which Cp max (T_{max}) is reached. It is therefore understood that these accidents occur following an accidental intravascular (arterial or venous) injection of local anaesthetics or following a slower systemic absorption of an extravascular volume of local anaesthetic.

The actual plasma concentration of local anaesthetic following loco-regional anaesthesia is challenging to predict and may be influenced by several factors (e.g., intrinsic drug properties, patient characteristics, site and mode of administration, etc.), as illustrated in Table 9.3 [32, 33].

Severe clinical manifestations of local anaesthetic toxicity may arise in patients with a right–left cardiac shunt, even at minimal intravascular drug concentrations, likely due to the *first-pass* pulmonary *uptake* effect of local anaesthetics. The clearance of amide local anaesthetics is closely linked to hepatic blood flow and liver function, meaning that proportionally higher plasma concentrations peaks will occur in patients with liver and/or heart failure, or during the use of drugs that inhibit hepatic metabolism (e.g., beta-blockers, H_2 antagonists). Renal insufficiency increases the volume of distribution of local anaesthetics and the accumulation of their metabolites.

The main clinical manifestation of neurological toxicity from local anaesthetics is convulsive seizures, which result from the inhibition of excitatory pathways in the amygdala. Most likely, this results either from an accidental intravascular injection or from rapid absorption at the injection site. Convulsions may be preceded by prodromal symptoms: confusion, agitation, dizziness, visual and auditory hallucinations, tinnitus, nystagmus, headache, paraesthesias and tingling in the extremities. As the concentration increases, tremors and fasciculations of the facial muscles and limbs may also manifest, up to generalized tonic–clonic grand mal seizure. With further increase in cerebral concentration, central nervous system depression up to coma, respiratory arrest may ensue. Generally, the convulsant concentration of a local anaesthetic is inversely proportional to the patient's partial pressure of CO_2 ($PaCO_2$): an increase in $PaCO_2$ or a decrease in pH results in a lowered seizure threshold, thereby enhancing the incidence of severe systemic toxicity [32, 33, 35].

The cardiovascular system is generally more resistant to the effects of local anaesthetics than the central nervous system. Neurological clinical manifestations of local anaesthetic toxicity typically occur at lower plasma concentrations than cardiovascular manifestations. This characteristic is defined by the *circulatory collapse/CNS excitation ratio*, which is a typical defining feature for each local anaesthetic. Specifically, bupivacaine exhibits a lower circulatory collapse/CNS excitation ratio compared to other less potent amide local anaesthetics (ropivacaine,

Table 9.3 Factors influencing the toxicity of local anaesthetics

Determinants of local anaesthesia toxicity:
• **Absorption** Local tissue perfusion; addition of vasoconstrictors Single shot vs multiple (or continuous infusion); administration site Injection Rate (velocity)
• **Patient characteristics/drug distribution** Weight and height; age Medical history, concomitant diseases and comorbidities; ongoing drug therapy Particular physiological condition (e.g. pregnancy)
• **Chemical and physical properties of local anaesthetic** Esteric or amideic nature of the local anaesthetic; half-life ($t_{½}$) pKa; liposolubility; proteins binding Distribution Volume (V_d)

levobupivacaine). The cardiotoxicity of local anaesthetics is plasma concentration-dependent and causes a depression of myocardial contractility with a decrease in cardiac output and profound hypotension. It may also cause alterations in intracardiac electrical conduction, responsible for sinus bradycardia, prolongation of PQ, QT and QRS complex intervals, atrio-ventricular block to asystole, arrhythmias due to re-entry phenomena resulting in supraventricular tachycardia, ventricular tachycardia or ventricular fibrillation. Local anesthetics have a biphasic action on peripheral vessel smooth muscle: at low plasma concentrations, local anaesthetics cause vasoconstriction; at higher concentrations, they decrease peripheral resistance; and at extremely high concentrations, they induce profound vasodilation via direct action on vascular smooth muscle [36]. If we follow the principle of the philosopher William of Ockham that it is pointless to seek more complex explanations when a simpler one works, the inhibition of sodium channels could be considered the primary mechanism underlying the cardiotoxicity of local anaesthetics. However, several studies indicate that local anaesthetics also interact with various other molecular targets, in addition to Na^+ channels, such as voltage-dependent potassium and calcium channels, HERG potassium channels, ATP-sensitive K^+ channels, NMDA receptors, β-adrenergic receptors, nicotinic receptors and G-protein-coupled K^+ and Ca^{2+} channels. The action of local anaesthetics at one or more of these sites of action may, therefore, contribute to their overall toxicity [37–42].

Several studies have demonstrated that bupivacaine has a narrower safety margin compared to ropivacaine, with levo-bupivacaine occupying an intermediate position. An *in vitro* study conducted on isolated rabbit hearts revealed that bupivacaine, levobupivacaine and ropivacaine all prolonged the QRS interval, with a 1:0.4:0.3 relative ratio [41].

In another study, *Santos* et al. [42] demonstrated that the cumulative dose of local anaesthetic required to induce convulsions and cardio-circulatory arrest in an experimental sheep model was lower for bupivacaine, followed by levobupivacaine, and the highest dose required for ropivacaine. However, the incidence of ventricular arrhythmias was similar in the three groups [34] (Table 9.4).

With regard to the treatment of severe complications, following systemic absorption of anaesthetic drugs, it should be noted that there is no specific antidote. A number of case reports [43–53], however, document the efficacy of lipid emulsion in the treatment of severe systemic toxicity, a potentially fatal complication. Severe acute toxicity from local anaesthetics is, in fact, often resistant to standard

Table 9.4 Relative toxicity of local anaesthetic drugs

Drug	CNS toxicity	Cardiotoxicity
Lidocaine	++	+
Mepivacaine	++	+
Prilocaine	++	±
Articaine	++	±
Bupivacaine	++++	++++++
Levobupivacaine (S)	+++	++++
S-Ropivacaine	+++	+++

resuscitative therapies due to the different molecular levels of action (cardiac ion channels, mitochondrial metabolism) of these substances [52, 54–57].

Although some studies conducted in experimental animal models suggest the superiority of lipid emulsion over epinephrine, vasopressin and their combination in the treatment of severe cardiotoxicity induced by local anaesthetic overdose, further researches are required in order to confirm the observations and, especially, to assess any clinical implications [58–62].

References

1. Govoni S, Cuzzocrea S, Lucchelli A, Navarra P, Racchi M, Scaglione F, Spampinato SM. Farmacologia. I edition. Zanichelli: Ambrosiana Publishing House; 2014.
2. Miller RD, Katzung BB. Local anaesthetics. In: Katzung BG, editor. General and clinical pharmacology. 5th English-language Italian edition. Piccin; 2003.
3. Narahashi T, Frazier DT, Yamada M. The site of action and active of local anaesthetics. Theory and pH experiments with tertialy compounds. J Pharmacol Exp Ther. 1970;171:32–44.
4. Winnie AP, LaVallee DA, Pesosa B, Masud ZK. Clinical pharmacokinetics of local anaesthetics. Can J Anaesth. 1977;24:252–5.
5. Tucker GT. Pharmacokinetics of local anaesthetics. Br J Anaesth. 1986;58:717–31.
6. Kaewjiaranai T, Srisatjaluk RL, Sakdajeyont W, Pairuchvej V, Wongsirichat N. The efficiency of topical anaesthetics as antimicrobial agents: a review of use in dentistry. J Dent Anesth Pain Med. 2018;18(4):223–33. https://doi.org/10.17245/jdapm.2018.18.4.223.
7. Parr AM, Zoutman DE, Davidson JS. Antimicrobial activity of lidocaine against bacteria associated with nosocomial wound infection. Ann Plast Surg. 1999;43(3):239–45. https://doi.org/10.1097/00000637-199909000-00003.
8. Stratford AF, Zoutman DE, Davidson JS. Effect of lidocaine and epinephrine on *Staphylococcus aureus* in a Guinea pig model of surgical wound infection. Plast Reconstr Surg. 2002;110:1275–9.
9. Reinertsen E, Sabayon M, Rice M, Lloyd M, Spektor B. Stellate ganglion blockade for treating refractory electrical storm: a historical cohort study. Can J Anaesth. 2021;68(11):1683–9. https://doi.org/10.1007/s12630-021-02068-1. English. Epub 2021 Jul 26
10. Savastano S, Dusi V, Baldi E, Rordorf R, Sanzo A, Camporotondo R, Fracchia R, Compagnoni S, Frigerio L, Oltrona Visconti L, De Ferrari GM. Anatomical-based percutaneous left stellate ganglion block in patients with drug-refractory electrical storm and structural heart disease: a single-Centre case series. Europace. 2021;23(4):581–6. https://doi.org/10.1093/europace/euaa319.
11. Sanghai S, Abbott NJ, Dewland TA, Henrikson CA, Elman MR, Wollenberg M, Ivie R, Gonzalez-Sotomayor J, Nazer B. Stellate ganglion blockade with continuous infusion versus single injection for treatment of ventricular arrhythmia storm. JACC Clin Electrophysiol. 2021;7(4):452–60. https://doi.org/10.1016/j.jacep.2020.09.032. *Epub 2020* Dec 24
12. Fudim M, Qadri YJ, Waldron NH, Boortz-Marx RL, Ganesh A, Patel CB, Podgoreanu MV, Sun AY, Milano CA, Tong BC, Harpole DH Jr, Mathew JP, Piccini JP. Stellate ganglion blockade for the treatment of refractory ventricular arrhythmias. JACC Clin Electrophysiol. 2020;6(5):562–71. https://doi.org/10.1016/j.jacep.2019.12.017. Epub 2020 Feb 26
13. Tian Y, Wittwer ED, Kapa S, McLeod CJ, Xiao P, Noseworthy PA, Mulpuru SK, Deshmukh AJ, Lee HC, Ackerman MJ, Asirvatham SJ, Munger TM, Liu XP, Friedman PA, Cha YM. Effective use of percutaneous stellate ganglion blockade in patients with electrical storm. Circ Arrhythm Electrophysiol. 2019;12(9):e007118. https://doi.org/10.1161/CIRCEP.118.007118. *Epub 2019* Sep 13

14. Prabhu MA, Prasad SBV, Abhilash SP, et al. Left sympathetic cardiac denervation in managing electrical storm: acute outcome and long term follow up. J Interv Card Electrophysiol. 2016;47:285–92. https://doi.org/10.1007/s10840-016-0153-2.
15. García-Morán E, Sliwinski-Herrera F, Cortes-Villar C, Sandín-Fuentes M, Pastor Báez G, San RA. Refractory electrical storm: a role for transient sympathetic blockade. Rev Esp Cardiol (Engl Ed). 2016;69(1):76–8. https://doi.org/10.1016/j.rec.2015.08.024. *Epub 2015* Dec 11
16. Amino M, Yoshioka K, Morita S, Otsuka H, Yamagiwa T, Umezawa K, Nakagawa Y, Yamamoto I, Hashida T, Ikari Y, Inokuchi S, Kodama I, Tanabe T. Is the combination therapy of IKr-channel blocker and left stellate ganglion block effective for intractable ventricular arrhythmia in a cardiopulmonary arrest patient? Cardiol J. 2007;14(4):355–65.
17. Nademanee K, Taylor R, Bailey WE, Rieders DE, Kosar EM. Treating electrical storm: sympathetic blockade versus advanced cardiac life support-guided therapy. Circulation. 2000;102(7):742–7. https://doi.org/10.1161/01.cir.102.742.
18. Gunduz OH, Kenis-Coskun O. Ganglion blocks as a treatment of pain: current perspectives. J Pain Res. 2017;10:2815–26. https://doi.org/10.2147/JPR.S134775. PMID: 29276402; PMCID: PMC573423
19. Yucel I, Demiraran Y, Ozturan K, Degirmenci E. Complex regional pain syndrome type I: efficacy of stellate ganglion blockade. J Orthop Traumatol. 2009;10(4):179–83.
20. Movafegh A, Razazian M, Hajimaohamadi F, Meysamie A. Dexamethasone added to lidocaine prolongs axillary brachial plexus blockade. Anesth Analg. 2006;102(1):263–7. https://doi.org/10.1213/01.ane.0000189055.06729.0a.
21. Foster HF, Anthony M, Levobupivacaine. A review of its pharmacology and use as a local anaesthetic. Drugs. 2000;59:551–79.
22. Kopacz DJ, et al. A comparison of epidural levobupivacaine 0.75% with racemic bupivacaine for lower abdominal surgery. Anesth Analg. 2000;90:642–8.
23. Cox CR, et al. Extradural S(−)bupivacaine: comparison with racemic RS-bupivacaine. Br J Anaesth. 1998;80:289–93.
24. Bader AM, et al. Clinical effects and maternal and fetal plasma concentrations of 0.5% epidural levobupivacaine versus bupivacaine for cesarean delivery. Anesthesiology. 1999;90:1596–601.
25. Glaser C, et al. Levobupivacaine versus racemic bupivacaine for spinal anaesthesia. Anesth Analg. 2002;94:194–8.
26. Burke D, et al. Comparison of 0.25% S(−)bupivacaine with 0.25% RS-bupivacaine for epidural analgesia in labour. Br J Anaesth. 1999;83:750–5.
27. Convery P, et al. Comparison of 0.125% levobupivacaine and 0.125% bupivacaine epidural infusions for labour analgesia [abstract]. Br J Anaesth. 1999;82(suppl.1):163.
28. Vercauteren MP, et al. Levobupivacaine combined with sufentanil and epinephrine for intrathecal labor analgesia: a comparison with racemic bupivacaine. Anesth Analg. 2001;93:996–1000.
29. Mulroy M. Systemic toxicity and cardiotoxicity from local anaesthetics: incidence and preventive measure. Reg Anesth Pain Med. 2002;27:556–61.
30. Auroy Y, Benhamou D, Bargues L, Ecoffey C, Falissard B, Mercier FJ, Bouaziz H, Samii k. Major complications of regional anaesthesia in France: the SOS regional anesthesia hotline service. Anesthesiology. 2002;97:1274–80.
31. Lee LA, et al. Complications associated with eye blocks and peripheral nerve blocks: an American society of anaesthesiologists closed claims analysis. Reg Anesth Pain Med. 2008;33(5):416–22.
32. Zink W, Graf BM. Toxikologie der Lokalanasthetika. Anaesthesist. 2003;52:1102–23.
33. Braid DP, Scott DP. The systemic absorption of local anaesthetic drugs. Acta Anaesthesiol Scand. 1996;(suppl 23):334–46.
34. Heavner JE. Cardiac toxicity of local anaesthetics in the intact isolated heart model: a review. Reg Anesth Pain Med. 2002;27(6):545–55.
35. Covino BG. Pharmacology of local anaesthetics agents. In: Rogers MC, Tinker JH, Covino BG, et al., editors. Principles and practice of anesthesiology. St. Louis: Mosby Year Book; 1993. p. 1235–57.
36. Blair MR. Cardiovascular pharmacology of local anaesthetics. Br J Anaesth. 1975;47:247–52.

37. Butterworth JF IV, Strichartz GR. Molecular mechanism of local anaesthesia: a review. Anesthesiology. 1990;72:711–34.
38. Hirota K, Browne T, Appadu BL, et al. Do local anaesthetics interact with dihydropyridine binding sites on neuronal L-type Ca^{2+} channels? Br J Anaesth. 1997;78:185–8.
39. Olschewski A, Olschewski H, Me B, et al. Effect of bupivacaine on ATP-dependent potassium channels in rat cardiomyocytes. Br J Anaesth. 1999;82:435–8.51
40. Sugimoto M, Uchida I, Fukami S, et al. The alpha and gamma subunit dependent effects of local anesthetics on recombinant GABA(A) receptors. Eur J Pharmacol. 2000;401:329–37.
41. Mazoit JX, Boico O, Samii K, et al. Myocardial uptake of bupivacaine: II. Pharmacokinetics and pharmacodynamics of bupivacaine enantiomers in the isolated perfused rabbit heart. Anesth Analg. 1993;77:477–82.
42. Santos AC, DeArmas P. Systemic toxicity of levobupivacaine, bupivacaine and ropivacaine during continuous intravenous infusion to nonpregnant and pregnant ewes. Anesthesiology. 2001;95:1256–64.
43. Foxall G, McCahon R, Lamb J, Hardman JG, Bedforth NM. Levobupivacaine-induced seizures and cardiovascular collapse treated with Intralipid. Anaesthesia. 2007;62:516–8.
44. Litz RJ, Popp SN, Koch T. Successful resuscitation of a patient with ropivacaine-induced asystole after axillary plexus block using lipid infusion. Anaesthesia. 2006;61:800–1.
45. Litz RJ, Roessel T, Heller AR, Stehr SN. Reversal of central nervous system and cardiac toxicity after local anaesthetic intoxication by lipid emulsion injection. Anesth Analg. 2008;106:1575–7.
46. Ludot H, Tharin JY, Belouadah M, Mazoit JX, Malinovsky JM. Successful resuscitation after ropivacaine and lidocaine-induced ventricular arrhythmia following posterior lumbar plexus block in a child. Anesth Analg. 2008;106:1572–4.
47. Smith HM, Jacob AK, Segura LG, Dilger JA, Torsher LC. Simulation education in anaesthesia training: a case report of successful resuscitation of 53 bupivacaine-induced cardiac arrest linked to recent simulation training. Anesth Analg. 2008;106:1581–4.
48. Warren JA, Thoma RB, Georgescu A, Shah SJ. Intravenous lipid infusion in the successful resuscitation of local anesthetic-induced cardiovascular collapse after supraclavicular brachial plexus block. Anesth Analg. 2008;106:1579–80.
49. McCutchen T, Gerancher JC. Early Intralipid therapy may have prevented bupivacaine-associated cardiac arrest. Reg Anaesth Pain Med. 2008;33(2):178–80.
50. Shah S, Gopalakrishnan S, Apuya J, Shah S, Martin T. Use of Intralipid in an infant with impending cardiovascular collapse due to local anaesthetic toxicity. J Anesth. 2009;23:439–41.
51. Marwick PC, Leven AI, Coetzee AR. Recurrence of cardiotoxicity after lipid rescue from bupivacaine- induced cardiac arrest. Anesth Analg. 2009;108:1344–6.
52. Zimmer C, Piepenbrink K, Riest G, Peters J. Cardiotoxic and neurotoxic effects after accidental intravascular bupivacaine administration: therapy with lidocaine propofol and lipid emulsion. Anaesthesist. 2007;56:449–53.
53. Spence AG. Lipid reversal of central nervous system symptoms of bupivacaine toxicity. Anesthesiology. 2007;107:515–7.
54. Castle NA. Bupivacaine inhibits the transient outward K^+ current but not the inward rectifier in rat ventricular myocytes. J Pharmacol Exp Ther. 1990;255:1038–46.
55. Clarkson CW, Hondeghem LM. Mechanism for bupivacaine depression of cardiac conduction: fast block of sodium channels during the action potential with slow recovery from block during diastole. Anaesthesiology. 1985;62:396–405.
56. Butterworth JFT, Brownlow RC, Leith JP, et al. Bupivacaine inhibits cyclic-3′,5′-adenosine monophosphate production. A possible contributing factor to cardiovascular toxicity. Anesthesiology. 1997;86:1112–9.
57. Reinikainem M, Hedman A, Pelkonen O, Ruokonen E. Cardiac arrest after interscalene brachial plexus block with ropivacaine and lidocaine. Acta Anaesthesiol Scand. 2003;47:904–6.
58. Heavner JE, Pitkanen MT, Shi B, Rosenberg PH. Resuscitation from bupivacaine-induced asystole in rats: comparison of different cardioactive drugs. Anesth Analg. 1995;80:1134–9.

59. Ohmura S, Kawada M, Ohta T, Yamamoto K, Kobayashi T. Systemic toxicity and resuscitation in bupivacaine-, levobupivacaine-, ropivacaine-infused rats. Anesth Analg. 2001;93:743–8.
60. Groban L, Deal DD, Vernon JC, James RL, Butterworth J. Cardiac resuscitation after incremental overdosage with lidocaine, bupivacaine, levobupivacaine and ropivacaine in anaesthetised dogs. Anesth Analg. 2001;92:37–43.
61. Mayr VD, Raedler C, Wenzel V, Lindner KH, Strohmenger HU. A comparison of epinephrine and vasopressin in a porcine model of cardiac arrest after rapid intravenous injection of bupivacaine. Anesth Analg. 2004;98:1426–31.
62. Mayr VD, Mitterschiffthaler L, Neurauter A, Gritsch C, Wenzel V, Muller T, Luckner G, Lindner KH, Strohmenger HU. A comparison of the combination of epinephrine and vasopressin with lipid emulsion in a porcine model of asphyxial cardiac arrest after intravenous injection of bupivacaine. Anesth Analg. 2008;106:1566–71.

Complications and Their Management 10

Enrico Baldi and Simone Savastano

Percutaneous stellate ganglion block (PSGB), like many medical procedures, may have some complications, but most of these, if treated by trained cardiologists, result in a minimum impact on the patient. All scientific studies reporting PSGB complications focused on outpatient procedures performed for antalgic purpose, not on the emergency setting of potentially lethal arrhythmias: in a Pain Management Division, even minor complications may cause inconveniences and be hardly tolerated by patients and clinicians, whereas in case of a potentially lethal condition, such as an electrical storm, they would produce a different response.

As described by Moore [1], who examined 2000 antalgic PSGBs, the complication rate of PSGB procedure is very low. More recent studies [2], based on surveys on about 45,000 PSGB, confirmed Moore's findings: 1.7 on 1000 PSGB interventions. In addition, adverse events, both in the anatomically guided and in the ultrasonography-guided approach, occur in equal amount [2].

PSGB complications can be classified considering either the phase of the procedure when they occur or the extent of effect they produce. The first comprehend technical (possible damages caused by the needle on anatomical structures), pharmacological (possible adverse effects of anaesthetics) and infectious damages (late-onset complications due to the contamination of the puncture site); the latter distinguish between local and systemic injuries.

Though with a very low frequency, haematoma is the local complication most reported in literature; it affects minor vessels, whereas it is extremely unlikely to affect the carotid artery that, in the anatomically guided approach, is dislocated, and

(translated by Chiara Barbaglia)

E. Baldi (✉) · S. Savastano
Division of Cardiology, Arrhythmology and Electrophysiology Unit, Fondazione IRCCS Policlinico San Matteo, Pavia, Italy
e-mail: enrico.baldi@unipv.it

S. Savastano (ed.), *Percutaneous Stellate Ganglion Block for Electrical Storm*,
https://doi.org/10.1007/978-3-031-81762-5_10

in the ultrasonography-guided procedure, can be clearly identified. Most haematomas were small and solved rapidly, but in very few cases, they required hospitalisation (n.b. collected data refer to outpatients undergoing antalgic PSGB therapy).

Elias M [3] discourages PSGB procedure in case of anticoagulant therapy for the risk of haemorrhage, yet, if we consider the aim and the context of the present study—an emergency cardiological setting—and the fact that most patients with heart disease receive either an acute or a chronic anticoagulant treatment, this complication should be overcome. Data show that in patients with antiplatelet or high levels of anticoagulation, as those undergoing extracorporeal membrane oxygenation (ECMO) and percutaneous coronary intervention (PCI), PSG block can be safely performed [4, 5]. Moreover, in a recent multicentre study [6] on 184 PSGBs, we reported no haemorrhagic complications despite the 86% of patients was under antiplatelet or anticoagulant therapy.

Hoarseness—caused by the anaesthesia of the recurrent laryngeal nerve—is reported in literature to occur in case of continuous percutaneous block owing to the high volume of anaesthetic, but it spontaneously regresses at the end of the procedure and continuous PSGB or the repetition of it need not be suspended.

Cough and dysphagia as well, reported among possible complications, are due to the temporary paresis of the recurrent laryngeal nerve.

In case the anaesthetic reached the brachial plexus, anaesthesia, hyposthenia or paresis of the ipsilateral arm can temporarily occur without any effect on the patient's life or health.

Paralysis of the phrenic nerve is among the rarest local adverse events of PSGB, but, should it occur bilaterally, it could produce a systemic effect; for this reason, Tian and colleagues, in their study on anti-arrhythmic PSGB, performed the intervention in intubated patients exclusively [7]. Fudim et al., instead, suggesting bilateral blockade can be safely performed in patients with spontaneous breathing, do not report this kind of complication [8].

Another possible, extremely rare, complication consists in the infection of the site of injection.

As to systemic complications, dizziness is one of the most common; artery hypertension, caused by the diffusion of the local anaesthetic into the carotid artery and consequent vagal blockade, can occur as well, though very seldom. Some, extremely rare, adverse events concerning the central nervous system comprehended convulsions, subdural or intraspinal blocks and even transient "locked-in" syndrome. Accidental injections of anaesthetic into the vertebral artery or into the subdural or subarachnoid space are the cause of such conditions. All the abovementioned adverse events solved, anyhow, in a short time—from 10 min to few hours depending on the kind of anaesthetic—with the complete neurological recovery of the patient and without any long- or mid-term effect.

Intra-vertebral injection or vertebral artery damage seem to be more frequent in the anatomically guided approach with Moore's technique and linked to the hyperextension of the neck and the consequent exposition of the vertebral artery and of the epidural space. For this reason, we suggest not to hyperextend the neck in order to minimize possible injuries.

In case of PSGB the occurrence of local anaesthetic systemic toxicity (LAST) must not be excluded, though extremely infrequent. It is difficult to predict the level of absorption of an anaesthetic, and the studies assessing its concentration after the block are few. In Hardy and colleagues [9], the plasmatic concentration of bupivacaine has always kept lower than the set toxicity limit (1.5–2 μg/ml), whereas in the paper by Wulf and colleagues, the concentration of bupivacaine exceeded the toxicity limit (2 μg/ml) only in 2% of cases [10].

Local anaesthetic systemic toxicity (LAST) leads to the excitation of the central nervous system (agitation, sensory changes and sudden psychiatric symptoms) followed by seizure activity and a depressive phase (drowsiness, coma and respiratory arrest); cardiac toxicity (hypertension, tachycardia, arrhythmias) or myocardial depression (bradycardia, hypotension, reduced myocardial contractility) may also occur. Prompt airway management by orotracheal intubation and subsequent administration of 20% intravenous lipid emulsion therapy (Table 10.1) are crucial to the treatment of LAST [10].

The promptness of administration of lipid emulsion is more important than the order of the kind of injection (bolus versus infusion), and if circulatory stability is not achieved by the above schedule, a new bolus or the increasing of the infusion to 0.5 mL/kg/min can be considered.

Administration of infusion should be continued for at least 10 minutes after patient's stability (recommended total dosage is 12 mL/kg).

In summary, complications in PSGB are connected to the possible interference with vascular structures or to a misplaced injection, yet they are extremely rare, and the suggestions illustrated in the present textbook can help reduce pitfalls to the minimum. Besides, the risks implied in PSGB are significantly fewer than the benefits for patients non-responding to standard medical treatments and at high risk of death. Furthermore, all other studies concerning PSGB treatment show that most patients who suffered an adverse event could anyhow undergo the planned therapeutic process.

In case of outpatient PSGB procedure, all studies recommend patient monitoring, venous access catheter, equipment for medical emergency and—as extra safety measure—anticonvulsants (i.e. short-acting benzodiazepines) for accidental intravascular injection.

Considering the life-saving purpose PSGB is performed for and the emergency setting this textbook refers to, if all the abovementioned recommendations are followed, the procedure is safe, and risks for patients are minimal. Left stellate ganglion block technique should become an essential skill in a cardiologist's training.

Table 10.1 Schedule for 20% intravenous lipid emulsion therapy for bolus and infusion

	Patient <70 kg	Patient >70 kg
Bolus	1.5 mL/kg in 2–3 min	100 mL in 2–3 min
Infusion	0.25 mL/kg/min	200–250 mL in 15–20 min

References

1. Moore DC. The anterior approach to the stellate ganglion. JAMA J Am Med Assoc. 1956;160(3):158. https://doi.org/10.1001/jama.1956.02960380006003.
2. Goel V, Patwardhan AM, Ibrahim M, Howe CL, Schultz DM, Shankar H. Complications associated with stellate ganglion nerve block: a systematic review. Reg Anesth Pain Med. 2019;44(6):669–78. https://doi.org/10.1136/rapm-2018-100127.
3. Elias M. Cervical sympathetic and stellate ganglion blocks. Pain Physician. 2000;3(3):294–304. https://doi.org/10.36076/ppj.2000/3/294.
4. Savastano S, Baldi E, Camporotondo R, Belliato M, Marinoni B, De Ferrari GM. Percutaneous stellate ganglion block and extracorporeal cardiopulmonary resuscitation: an effective and safe combination for refractory ventricular fibrillation. Europace. 2020;22(1):148. https://doi.org/10.1093/europace/euz180.
5. Savastano S, Dusi V, Baldi E, et al. Anatomical-based percutaneous left stellate ganglion block in patients with drug-refractory electrical storm and structural heart disease: a single-centre case series. Europace. 2021;23(4):581–6. https://doi.org/10.1093/europace/euaa319.
6. Savastano S, Baldi E, Compagnoni S, et al. Electrical storm treatment by percutaneous stellate ganglion block: the STAR study. Eur Heart J. 2024;45(10):823–33. https://doi.org/10.1093/eurheartj/ehae021.
7. Tian Y, Wittwer ED, Kapa S, et al. Effective use of percutaneous stellate ganglion blockade in patients with electrical storm. Circ Arrhythm Electrophysiol. 2019;12(9):e007118. https://doi.org/10.1161/CIRCEP.118.007118.
8. Fudim M, Qadri YJ, Waldron NH, et al. Stellate ganglion blockade for the treatment of refractory ventricular arrhythmias. JACC Clin Electrophysiol. 2020;6(5):562–71. https://doi.org/10.1016/j.jacep.2019.12.017.
9. Hardy PAJ, Williams NE. Plasma concentrations of bupivacaine after stellate ganglion block using two volumes of 0.25% bupivacaine plain solution. Br J Anaesth. 1990;65(2):243–4. https://doi.org/10.1093/bja/65.2.243.
10. Wulf H, Maier C, Schele HA, Wabbel W. Plasma concentration of bupivacaine after stellate ganglion blockade. Anesth Analg. 1991;72(4):546–8. https://doi.org/10.1213/00000539-199104000-00022.

Correction to: Efficacy and Safety Data

S. Savastano, Francesca Romana Gentile,
and Sara Compagnoni

Correction to:
Chapter 5 in: S. Savastano (ed.), *Percutaneous Stellate Ganglion Block for Electrical Storm*, https://doi.org/10.1007/978-3-031-81762-5_5

The correction to the author's name was inadvertently missed in the chapter. The author's name has been changed from "Romana Gentile" to "Francesca Romana Gentile."

The updated version of this chapter can be found at
https://doi.org/10.1007/978-3-031-81762-5_5

S. Savastano (ed.), *Percutaneous Stellate Ganglion Block for Electrical Storm*,
https://doi.org/10.1007/978-3-031-81762-5_11

MIX
Papier aus verantwortungsvollen Quellen
Paper from responsible sources
FSC® C105338
FSC
www.fsc.org

If you have any concerns about our products,
you can contact us on
ProductSafety@springernature.com

In case Publisher is established outside the EU,
the EU authorized representative is:
Springer Nature Customer Service Center GmbH
Europaplatz 3, 69115 Heidelberg, Germany

Printed by Libri Plureos GmbH
in Hamburg, Germany